PRAISE FOR JENNA MINECCI

"Jenna is a great trainer to work with. After experiencing four knee surgeries, I was extremely hesitant about training for fear of reinjury. As a trainer myself, it's hard to admit but sometimes we can all use a little help to get back on track. Jenna is very knowledgeable when it comes to knee anatomy and I knew I could trust her cues, and count on her to know if it was okay to work through some discomfort or if we needed to back off completely. After just two months of working with Jenna, I became pain free for the first time in years and happily enjoy demoing my boot camp workouts to my classes again! Having someone right there focused solely on your progress is worth every penny! I highly recommended her!" *Kim Liles-Personal Trainer, Fitness Instructor*

"In today's healthcare marketplace, there has never been a better time to consider a having expert guidance through your ACL injury and recovery process. I have known Jenna for 10 years going back to the days when she was my patient recovering from Orthopedic surgery. She was very focused on her own Rehab as she recovered from injuries as an athlete and with that focus grew her passion and dedication to change the lives of others with pain and injuries. It wasn't soon after her first surgery that she was

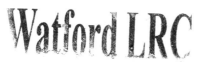

interning with me (at the age of 15!) so that she could start to learn as much as possible about rehabilitation and the human body.

She is extremely knowledgeable in the area of Kinesiology and Exercise Science and because of her past experiences she is an excellent choice to guide you through a complete recovery. Without any hesitation I recommend Jenna to any of my patients who need a Preventative ACL Training Program or extra guidance with Post Rehabilitation Programs designed to enhance your ACL reconstruction recovery." *Terry Trundle-ATC, LAT, PTA Athletic Rehab Institute- Owner/Director of Sports Medicine*

"Running has been an important part of my life since my first marathon in 1996. When I injured my knee, in May of 2015, and could not run; I was not a happy camper! I went to the orthopedist, and he x-rayed both knees, and said that I had cartilage, but the tendons, muscles, etc. were extremely inflamed. He advised me to stop running and initiate a program of exercise therapy to help heal the knee. Jenna built a customized program of home and in-the-gym exercises, and began working with me three times per week.

Within three months, my knees were feeling great! Now I can run again, and I will continue the exercises for probably the rest of my life to ensure strong muscles and tendons, and flexibility to enable me to exercise and run. I have already signed up for my next half marathon which I thought I could never do again! Yay for Jenna and a great program!" ***Carol Johnson-Runner for life***

"I am Harland Gunn. I am an ex-NFL football player. I spent the majority of my NFL career with The Atlanta Falcons. While preparing during the offseason with The Falcons, I wanted to tend to my chronic issues of hip mobility and core instability. I knew I had issues with my core not being as strong as I'd like, and my hips being rigid from squatting heavy weights throughout my football career. The hip pain was limiting my performance.

After a month of consistent work outs, mobility work, and stretching with Jenna, my hip issues were considerably reduced and I felt extremely free moving around during football practices and performing everyday tasks. My core strength was significantly improved and I was quicker coming up off the line. If I were to come across younger football players dealing with similar issues, I would refer them to Jenna to have their functional movement issues tended to. Thanks again Jenna." ***Harland Gunn-Former NFL Offensive Lineman***

"Before I started working with Jenna I had a lot of knee problems if I played tennis more than twice a week. After just a few months with Jenna I was able to go to a week-long tennis clinic and I didn't have any knee pain at all!

Jenna helped me see that my knee pain was a combination of knee, hamstring, and hip issues, and she used weight training, stretching, and other exercises to address them. I'm very thankful for Jenna and I can't wait to see what we accomplish next." *Kyle Barry-enjoys tennis and staying active*

"We crossed paths on Instagram by her simply reaching out and being supportive, but the bond we have now is unbreakable. I cannot thank Jenna enough for being my rock that I can lean on. I've blown up her phone so many times, yet not once has she shut me out or not replied. No one believed there was something else wrong with my previous ACL reconstructed knee until Jenna helped me talk through and diagnose my injury from my symptoms, X Rays, surgery scribe notes, and MRIs.

My coaches and even my surgeon didn't believe me but she did and she determined what was wrong before my surgeon. She is always thorough and honest with her replies and I greatly appreciate that. She's a great role model and I aspire to be just like her. She is changing the lives of young adults one at a time and she's doing it well!! We need more people like Jenna out there! Our paths definitely crossed for a reason and I'm so grateful for it. Our journeys are not over just yet but I take great comfort in knowing that we will always have each other's backs (or should I say knee's...!) I LOVE YOU JENNA!" *Sarfina Seretharan-Golfer at Marshall University*

"As a lifelong competitive athlete (soccer, martial art and gymnastics) and a full time martial art professional with more than 30 years of martial art training under my 'wheels' (a.k.a. knees), Jenna's approach to heal, train and strengthen provided the best formula for my recent recovery from a medial posterior meniscus tear on my right knee. In 2009, I suffered the same injury on my left knee and underwent a surgery to remove the torn portion to regain full function, reduce pain and swelling. I wish I knew then what I know now...and more importantly I wish I knew Jenna!

Although the 2009 surgery successfully removed the primary discomfort, returned the majority of my range of motion and allowed me to resume regular activity the full range of motion took nearly six months to return to the left leg. Subsequently in 2010 (nearly twelve months after the meniscus surgery) I fractured the navicular in my right foot, which was not recommended for surgery. Prior to working with Jenna no other doctor or therapist I've worked with in past rehab sessions noticed the misalignment from my right foot injury and how it may be affecting my performance.

The first question Jenna asked during her initial diagnosis/assessment when we began our first session was about my right foot. As a result, she immediately began to work foot strength and balance exercises into my right knee rehabilitation program. Over an eight-week period Jenna not only challenged me and educated me in ways that helped me better understand the mechanics of my injury, but also provided a phased approach to strengthen the areas around my injured meniscus.

At the conclusion of the eight-week training period, I was not only able to participate fully in a martial art demonstration I had been preparing for overall for twelve years (more intensely over the last eight weeks), but also deliver a full performance over a four-day period of a combined 16 hours of training. I can confidently say if I knew in 2009 what and who I know now, I would not have chosen surgery over the rehabilitation and strength program Jenna personally designed for my full recovery! Thank you, Jenna, for helping me and keeping me on the path to full range, pain free, and functional strength!" *Mr. Sule K. Welch, President/Founder/Sifu/Head Coach, The Welch Martial Art Experience - Fitness Concepts Empowering Life®*

SURVIVING 7

THE EXPERT'S GUIDE TO ACL SURGERY: RECOVERY, REHABILITATION, AND PREVENTION

JENNA MINECCI

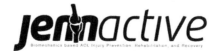

Biomechanics based ACL Injury Prevention, Rehabilitation, and Recovery

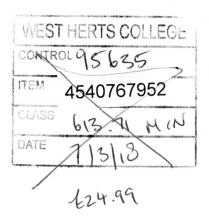
ISBN-10: 0999493833

ISBN-13: 978-0999493830

CONTENTS

FOREWORD

I have known Jenna for many years as she became my patient almost 12 years ago. I have treated many post-operative ACL patients in my long career in Sports Physical Therapy and Athletic Training. No one has been as dedicated to their rehabilitation goals as Jenna. After many knee surgeries, she continues to be one of the most focused patients I have ever seen. I know her efforts and intensity in the uncertainty facing her will be met with grace and personal faith of doing the right thing.

No matter the challenge of multiple surgeries, as she contemplates future procedures to be performed on her knee, she still has the self-discipline and integrity to face her recovery. Her knowledge level is exceptional. Jenna has a high level of experience in exercise science, biomechanics and human performance. Her specialty in post-therapy extended care has allowed her to help many people reach their functional goals. She is also interested in expanding her knowledge in the prevention of ACL injuries.

Her personal experiences while surviving seven surgeries has provided her the opportunity to write her "Story." Sharing the content of this book will encourage many patients who may be facing ACL reconstruction.

At the end of the day Jenna always knows what her goals are. I am proud to be her rehabilitation consultant, fellow Tennessee Vols fan but most of all just being a good friend with common goals.

> ***Terry Trundle ATC, LAT, PTA***
> ***Owner of Athletic Rehab Institute***
> ***Rehab Consultant for BenchMark***
> ***Physical Therapy***
> ***Acworth, Georgia***

INTRODUCTION

This isn't a book meant to be only about my story; it is a guide for what I wish I had known at the beginning of my journey when I tore my ACL the first time. As a thirteen-year-old determined soccer player my biggest priority and focus was returning to the soccer field quickly. I wasn't concerned with how this injury would affect me in 10 years or 30 years. I wasn't thinking about my risks associated with subsequent injuries. I didn't know the importance of finding, interviewing, and having an open and working relationship with my surgeon. I wanted to get better so I could be a soccer player again. I wanted to get better so I could be active and normal again. Most athletes have the same focus. We find a surgeon, have surgery, and work on returning to sport.

It's a simple process and ACL injuries are becoming so common we truly believe we will return to our sport and everything will be exactly as it was before the injury. The reality is this injury is not as simple and clean cut as we make it out to be. And ACL reconstructions are still not being performed as an A+ procedure. Many athletes do not return to sport at all and even more athletes require multiple revision surgeries because of poor surgical techniques, inadequate rehabilitation, returning to sport too soon, failed cadaver grafts, and a host of other reasons. Now that you have torn your ACL, your life is forever changed. Your knees will have increased risk of meniscus tears, arthritis, and re-injury forever, no matter who your surgeon is, no matter how hard you rehabilitate, no matter how dedicated you are. ACL injury doesn't care who you are and how badly you want to overcome it. The things I wish I had known after my first injury can help you to withstand many of the obstacles now standing in front of the athletic life you know and love. Fighting to maintain your athletic and active life is of utmost priority so prepare yourself of the recovery journey that will last a lifetime.

1

THE INJURY

In elementary school, I was always on a mission to prove something. Most of my time was spent singing boy band lyrics with my best girl friend or playing any type of sport imaginable with the boys in my neighborhood. We played football, flashlight tag, sharks and minnows, basketball, biking, war, and would even make up our own combinations of sports. I had a small chip on my shoulder. I always wanted to prove I was just as good as the boys were. At recess one day, I finally realized my strength. Besides being great at catching a football, which as a girl wouldn't get me anywhere, I learned I could kick. I kicked a home run after being chosen last in a pick-up game of kickball. I felt invincible when kicking the ball. It was a skill that gave me recognition at recess in elementary school and made me feel important and accepted by my peers. A cute boy became one of my new friends and began to mentor me and build up my soccer skills and confidence until he finally convinced me to join a soccer team. Being part of a sports team was incredible. I was very competitive and this fueled my need for excellence even more. After a few years of playing and having a blast, I finally made the commitment to join a more competitive league. It was 2004, I was 14-years-old and I had just joined my first select soccer team. I was ecstatic and determined to work hard and become a great player. We played year-round and we traveled to regional tournaments. Soccer became my life and my biggest goal was to play on the high school soccer team and go on to play college soccer at my mom's Alma Mater, the University of Tennessee.

That first season came to an end and we were at our State Cup tournament. Our goalie was injured and when the coach asked me to sub in as goalie because he knew I could catch the ball, I was flattered. I stepped right in and after ten minutes of him coaching me on techniques I was ready. He told me to be aggressive and if someone dribbled the ball into the box I should challenge them head on which would minimize the angle for the shooter to score. Without hesitation, I did exactly that. The forward entered the goalie box and I charged, diving for the ball and closed my eyes as I collided into her. I stole the ball and this sudden rush of exciting emotions filled me up. But almost as instantly as my excitement emerged, I also felt a sharp, pinching, stabbing pain in my knee. I thought nothing of it and stood up to punt the ball back out to my teammates. The ball hit my kicking foot and flopped to the floor like a pancake. Coach screamed in fury and I was frozen. Not from embarrassment but from pain. I flagged at the coach to get me out of the game but he didn't understand that I was hurt and became instantly distracted following the ball to the other side of the field. There were only about ten minutes left in the game so I decided to tough it out and be there for my team because they needed a goalie. I told my defense that something was wrong and I needed their back-up, and as luck would have it, the ball didn't come to me the rest of the game.

I hobbled to the center of the field to shake everyone's hands and Coach yelled at me for limping. We had won the tournament and the entire team went out for celebratory ice cream! I staggered to the car assuring myself and my father that it was just a little twist and it would feel better soon. By the time we made it to the ice cream parlor ten minutes later my knee had quadrupled in size. My dad had to carry me inside. On Monday morning, I went to school on a pair of crutches that my neighbor lent me. I had just started my freshman year of high school and getting on and off the school bus on crutches was extremely difficult and embarrassing. After a few days, my pain subsided and I stopped using my crutches. I noticed my knee felt different. It didn't hurt but it just felt weak and unstable. I figured those symptoms would eventually subside so I continued about my normal life. One day, getting off the school bus with those large stairs, my knee buckled under me and I toppled down the stairs landing on the street next to the school bus. As a new little freshman, this was extremely embarrassing and to make matters worse, the juniors in the back of the bus starting laughing, pointing at me, and making fun of me for being a klutz. I did my best to walk the rest of the way home but I could feel something wasn't right. A few days later, I was emptying the dishwasher, one of my nightly chores, and as I turned to grab a plate from the dishwasher and pivoted to place it up into the cabinet my knee buckled underneath me and I accidentally dropped the plate. It went crashing down onto the floor and shattered. I caught myself before falling but told my mom I needed help. Something didn't feel right.

We scheduled an appointment with an orthopedic surgeon very close to our house. It was a very large practice with different surgeons of different specialties. I was terrified. Why did we have to see a surgeon? My mom explained to me this doctor was specialized in sports injuries but not to worry because we just need to find out what is wrong with my knee. After talking to nurses and physician' assistants we patiently waited for the doctor to see me. Suddenly, he walked into the room chuckling a little bit. After examining my knee very quickly he told me my ACL was torn and I needed an MRI and surgery. He exclaimed, "Don't worry, the guy next door had ACL surgery with me last year, and he just came back in with a torn ACL on the other knee!" I looked at my mom. I wasn't even sure what to think. I was trying to understand what ACL surgery meant and why I needed surgery. And then I began wondering how likely this could be for me to end up like the man in the room next door, and why the doctor seemed amused at this information?

ACL surgery? What is an ACL, and why do I need one? Surgery with almost a year-long recovery; how was I going to do it? And what is this doctor talking about, a man coming to see him with a second ACL tear? How can this be possible? I was extremely upset. I was at a new school and hadn't made a lot of friends yet; I just knew that joining the soccer team would help me meet new friends and would be so much fun. It turned out the first available surgery date was on the same exact day as soccer tryouts.

At first I was angry, upset, and annoyed. Why me? Why do all the other girls get to try out for the soccer team and I must have surgery? Why couldn't this have happened to someone else or later in the year after I had at least joined the team? What was I going to do? In the moment, it hit me. I still want to play soccer. There will still be a tryout next year. I decided I was going to do everything in my power to recover, rehabilitate, and comeback from this surgery as a better athlete than before and I was going to try out and make the high school soccer team! As soon as I came back to school after my surgery, I crutched into the JV soccer coach's classroom and announced to her my mission and my dedication to my high school soccer team and that I wanted to be a part of it even without the use of my leg. I enlisted to be the team manager. The position was not exactly what I had expected; there were some fun leadership roles but for the most part I was cleaning up after practice and shagging balls for all the girls while on my crutches and then limping around with my knee brace. It was not ideal but I was part of the team and that was worth it.

Rehabilitation was grueling. I went to a physical therapy office down the street from my high school so my mom had time to take me and still get me to school before starting her own work day. I was excited to work hard in order to recover but sometimes I felt very alone in the process. Most of my peers were playing sports and couldn't relate to my life or the recovery road ahead of me. It hurt me a lot to hear girls on the soccer team complaining about going to practice. I thought I wish I was healthy enough to even play! My physical therapist was juggling three or four patients at a time and I hardly knew what I was supposed to be doing. As I started to progress and stopped wearing a knee brace, my physical therapist actually had to ask me which knee was the injured one. I absolutely couldn't believe he wouldn't know which knee was injured after all the months I had been strengthening my right leg with him. Very soon after, my insurance visits ran out and I was discharged from physical therapy. I was only about three or four months out of my surgery; we hadn't started running yet or even doing any heavy strength training. It seemed odd to me that I could be finished with rehab already but the therapist told me to take things slow and that I was on my own now.

I taught myself how to run again and I started running everywhere. I would run every day when I got home from school because I knew I had such a long way to go to get back in shape before next year's soccer tryouts. I wasn't as strong as I used to be and running hurt me a lot of the time but I just shrugged it off and told myself I would progress and it would all be fine. I began going to the local elementary school four days per week after school to practice ball handling skills and running sprints. I had good days and bad days. Some days I felt halfway normal again and other days I felt like I could barely make use of my legs. It was like I had all of these fancy moves in my head and as I relayed the signals down to my legs somehow the signal got lost. I felt helpless but again I blamed it on the surgery and kept pushing forward.

By the fall of my sophomore year in high school, I was

about eight-months out from ACL surgery on my right knee. I knew I wasn't even close to the level I used to play at and I knew that meant I couldn't keep up with my old select soccer team. I reluctantly joined a rec league thinking that any competition is competition and maybe it would help me to progress and prepare for high school tryouts in the spring. It was great! I was playing again! I felt invincible, unstoppable, and elated to play. I was a normal soccer player again! It was everything I had missed for so long while I was injured and I was so happy to be back in action. But deep inside my tough, determined exterior a small part of me was terrified to tear my ACL again. It happened so fast the first time and it still seemed so fresh despite my yearlong recovery. I didn't share those feelings with anyone else because I was scared saying them aloud would make it a reality. I still had a blast playing soccer again and the fall season flew by. I continued my daily runs, ball handling drills, and sprints. My focus was on the high school soccer tryouts and even the fear inside me wasn't going to stand in my way of accomplishing this dream. Spring season was fast approaching and I continued to play on the same rec team because I needed playing time to get back to being 100%.

Before I knew it, it was time for high school soccer tryouts. I was ready and I had worked so hard to get there. Tryouts were not exactly what I had expected. All of the girls from the freshmen team were trying out again, of course, but the coaches didn't seem to even be paying attention. They were treating it almost like a practice and any time I had a drill or touched the ball it seemed they weren't even watching. The next day they posted the team on the locker room door. My palms were sweating as I read the list of names. I wasn't on the list. They had chosen every single girl from last year and that was it. All the work I had done flashed into my eyes in a moment of grief, disgust, and outrage. I can't believe they didn't notice me or all the hard work I had done. I didn't want to be left with nothing after all of that, so I halfheartedly joined the track team.

Track was not the same. I hated running. I treasured running when I knew I was training for the sport I loved but running for nothing wasn't exactly as motivating. One day at track practice the soccer coach was walking around and talking with some of the athletes. I ran the 100m and 200m while he was standing there and was, of course, wearing my soccer gear because that is all I owned. He walked right up to me and announced I was fast and he didn't understand why I hadn't tried out for the soccer team. My stomach fell to the floor. I couldn't believe what he just said. That was my biggest dream. I explained to him that I was the girl in the knee brace and he quickly remembered and told me he was sorry for my injury and walked away. It hit me; I was never going to be the same after that and no one was going to think of me as the same either. But the state soccer tournament was that weekend and my rec team needed me. I headed to soccer practice after school later that afternoon.

Practice was very easy that day because coach didn't want to wear us out before the tournament in a few days. He had us warm up, work on ball handling drills, and then he let us just play for fun. My friends and I were excited and starting acting out our plays as we did them, almost like we were our own announcers. "Jenna has the ball! She dribbles down the right field and veers over into the corner! She has the perfect setup with two girls open in front of the goal! And..." I planted my left foot to kick the ball with my right and it happened. I knew instantly what it was and what had happened. I was in such disbelief that I laid there face down laughing. Did this really just happen to me again? Is this on my good knee? I don't have a good knee anymore? Are you kidding me?! I didn't get back up, I couldn't.

Pain started to irradiate from my knee to my entire body. I began to sweat, shake, and it felt like time had frozen and turned into super slow motion. Coach ran up to me and I was in such shock that I wasn't able to tell him I knew I had torn my ACL. Even worse, I knew I had torn my ACL on my good knee days before the state cup where my team needed me. I don't think I had managed to say anything yet but he knew something was wrong by the look on my face and desperately pleaded for a doctor. Surprisingly there was a doctor on the field and he quickly came over to help. The doctor and my coach told me to stand up and I was finally able to speak. "No", I mumbled. "I can't walk. I can't put pressure on it or I will fall right back down again. Are you going to catch me?"

They said I was overreacting and they would catch me if I fell. Reluctantly I placed my left leg in front of me to take a step and sure enough my entire leg buckled underneath me and I fell to the ground. They did not catch me. But they quickly realized I wasn't faking it and carried me to the side of the field. I instructed them to lay me on the side of the field where there was a hill so I could begin to elevate my knee before the swelling took over and instructed someone to call my mom and bring my crutches. I knew what my diagnosis was, I could just feel it. I knew what journey was ahead of me and how difficult it would be. I knew nothing I could do could change any of this and I felt so helpless. I just laid there looking at the sky thinking...There must be a solution. This happened way too easily to be uncommon. There has to be a way to prevent this and a better way to treat these injuries after they happen.

My pain was a lot worse this time. I kept thinking maybe my leg was broken. Maybe that's why it hurt more. Maybe it isn't my ACL and it's just a leg break. That would be okay. That wouldn't be as bad. My mom got to the field and I was shaking. She asked why I was shaking and all I said was "it's from the pain." We knew what was in front of me and there was no reason to go to the emergency room when we just needed to see my surgeon. She drove me home and we stopped at Steak-N-Shake for a banana milkshake. I told her in that drive through line that I wanted to change the world of knees!

It turns out I tore my ACL, MCL, and meniscus which would explain the increased pain levels. I had surgery and began the long road to recovery again. But this time it didn't go as well as planned. I wasn't progressing quickly enough and everything I did was very painful. My surgeon had no explanation for me so he sent me for a second opinion to a very highly regarded athletic trainer in Atlanta. I didn't know it at the time but this would change my life forever.

After my first visit with Terry Trundle I knew he was different than the rest. He was extremely knowledgeable and loved to talk so I learned a plethora of information just in one visit and he was a Tennessee graduate; something was meant to be. But he didn't bring good news. Unfortunately, because of the lack of stability in both of my knees Terry had to refer me to another surgeon. After MRIs, and many long talks with the new surgeon and Terry, it was decided that the first surgeon didn't do the most appropriate placement for my ACL in both of my knees which created a large degree of laxity. This basically means my knees were way too loose to be functional and if I wanted to decrease my pain and lead a somewhat active life I needed a revision surgery on both of my knees.

I couldn't believe it. How could this happen? I had already endured an invasive surgery on both of my knees but now I had to do them both again. My athletic career was over and I had only just turned 15. I wouldn't be able to play high school soccer and I certainly wouldn't be skilled enough to become a Lady Volunteer on the University of Tennessee's soccer team. But I had to do it anyway. As much pain as it would cause and as much time as it would consume from my normal high school life; both surgeries had to be done in order to preserve the integrity of my knees.

We discussed our surgery options. This time, approaching my second ACL surgery on each knee, I began to question my new surgeon more. Because I had a Patella Tendon graft for my first surgeries on each knee, my surgeon explained to me it would be much easier to use a cadaver graft for my next ACL surgery on each knee. He said there wasn't any of my own tissue left to harvest (which I later found out was not true) and using a cadaver would make for an easier recovery process. A cadaver, you mean a dead person? Where do you find this dead person? How do we know they were healthy and disease free? How on earth is a dead person's tissue going to help my knee heal? Does the graft arrive in a FedEx envelope and if so, why is the one for me? Do you wash it? Does it smell? I couldn't bear the thought of some dead person's tissue inside of me so I just trusted my surgeon and tried my best not to think about it.

We carefully planned each surgery and which knee was the most symptomatic so we could operate on it first. It was a huge risk because each knee was very loose so whichever knee we chose, we still had to hope I was strong enough on the other knee in order to navigate on crutches and get to high school, and my after school job.

The biggest blessing in all of this was spending so much time with Terry during my rehab. He genuinely cared about my well-being and he started to teach me why we were doing what we were doing and why it was so important. It all just clicked for me. I realized how amazing and resilient the human body is and understand there had to be a better way to approach ACL injuries and surgeries. There had to be a better quality of care than the surgeon who put both of my ACLs in at the wrong angle or the physical therapist who didn't even remember which leg I had injured. These are devastating sometimes career ending injuries and surgeries and no one was taking it seriously enough, except for Terry.

I decided to become an intern for Terry because I already spent so much time there and I had such a huge desire for functional knowledge of the human body and its biomechanics. I realized my dream of playing soccer was over but if I learned everything about the human body, rehabilitation, and the ACL, I could make a difference one day. I was going to execute my mission on changing the world of knees and I wanted to start now.

One and a half years later I arrived in the parking lot of Terry's physical therapy office. I was a senior in high school with high hopes to attend the University of Tennessee and major in Kinesiology. I had met with the head of the Exercise Science and Kinesiology major at age 16 to assure this choice in majors would be good for my goal of changing the world of knees. I had known what I wanted for a long time. I started crutching my way to the front door of the physical therapy office and I received an email on my phone. After entering the office and crutching over to Terry I checked my email before starting my shift. I had been accepted to the University of Tennessee!!!!! I couldn't believe I got accepted and I couldn't believe I found out while I was with Terry another Tennessee graduate and my mentor. It was meant to be!! We started dancing and crutch dancing around the office singing Rocky Top! It was pure joy.

By the time high school ended I had gone through five surgeries. Two were from the first initial ACL injuries, two were the ACL revision surgeries, and one was a hip surgery that probably was injured at the same time as one of my ACL injuries. I had attended a few homecoming dances, proms, ran the flags at the football games, and graduation - all on crutches, in a knee brace, or both. It was difficult struggling to fit in with my peers while no one understood why I continued to have surgery after surgery. I'm sure many of the people who didn't know me thought I was crazy and assumed I kept getting injured playing soccer which was not the case. Sometimes I would go a semester without seeing certain kids at my school and when we changed schedules and has classes together again they would be shocked I was still on crutches with a huge knee brace. Some people would ask what was taking so long and then I would explain it was different surgeries. No one understood. I was very shy in high school and the constant attention my crutches and injuries gave me was very uncomfortable. Some of the guys in my classes would make fun of me or mess with my crutches by changing the height levels or move them across the room so I couldn't get to them when the bell rang for class changes. Only one of the teachers even stood up for me. My history teacher noticed and called the boys out on their childish antics but it didn't stop them.

It is very ironic though, eventually all three of those boys tore their ACL or broke their leg, requiring them to be on crutches and injured too. I will never forget, when we were practicing for high school graduation, I had just starting walking again after my 4th ACL surgery. I was very slow and still had a little bit of a hobble. We practiced our line up and walking sequences in that large auditorium for what felt like hours. My knee started getting extremely tired. We practiced one final walk through which required us to walk from our seats, up the stairs, across the stage, down the stairs, and exit the building. I was so tired and starting getting slower and slower with my walking. My last name began with the letter M and suddenly the teacher screamed out, "Why is the last half of the alphabet going so slow!?" I was so embarrassed and exhausted I almost cried. I was holding up half of our graduating class. That is over 250 people! What if this happens tomorrow at graduation?

Maybe I shouldn't go to graduation. I was so nervous and upset. Thankfully one guy in my class defended me by telling our teacher I was injured and it wasn't my fault. I couldn't believe one of the same guys who was making fun of me in classes stood up and defended me to our teacher in front of our entire graduating class. I was truly touched and thankful for his understanding and help.

I left for college with the goal in mind that I would change the world of knees and I would learn as much as I could about gaining strength and function to the lower extremities so I could overcome my setbacks and help other young girls to do the same. While in one of my first classes in my Kinesiology major at the University of Tennessee, we discussed possible career paths in the field and how to sign up for internship programs in order to gain experience. The first internship program on the PowerPoint slide was an internship with the Lady Volunteer Sports Medicine Staff. I couldn't believe I could be a part of something that amazing! I could still be a Lady Vol! I wrote down the contact information and quickly sent my resume after class. Working with the athletes was such a rewarding experience and the Athletic Trainers who supervised the undergraduates were extremely knowledgeable. I learned so much and most importantly I got to help many athletes with nagging injuries. There were even a few ACL surgeries and rehabilitations.

I also became certified as a personal trainer and began training at a local gym in order to help pay the bills. I never thought I would stick with it but I began to realize I was great at being a personal trainer. My clients all had knee or low back pain and by using the knowledge I had learned from Terry in high school and with the Lady Vols Sports Medicine team in college, I quickly became the go to trainer for weight loss and decreasing pain. Unfortunately, before college was over I had to have another knee surgery. This was due to a personal training manager who pushed me too far. I should have told him I wasn't strong enough to perform the move he wanted me to try but his yelling intimidated me and I didn't want to look like the weak trainer. In retrospect, my injury was more of a result of trying to perform that hard exercise with a nonfunctional ACL graft, although I didn't know it at the time. The surgeon had no explanation for my insane amount of pain and instability because the MRI revealed a normal ACL with no tears but decided to operate on me anyway. He performed a meniscectomy and a scope but couldn't figure out why I was in pain. With this most recent surgery and reoccurring pain and weakness, it was very hard for me to gain confidence as a beginner trainer because I was worried about my knees slowing me down or holding me back.

I wasn't as fit as some of the trainers who were body builders and that made me self-conscious because I would look at my knees as a limiting factor. With experience and maturity, I learned I had the power to change my thoughts and to eliminate negative feelings. I realized I could better relate with my clients and cared more about their injuries because I knew what experiencing chronic pain was like. Despite my newly found confidence in my knowledge and abilities, I was still turned down for an exciting job working with NCAA and professional athletes because I could not perform some of the complex drills and exercises required for the job. This broke my heart and partially made me give up because I knew I had the knowledge and expertise to excel with that company but I put my head down and focused. Excuses and limitations weren't going to help me find my dream job. Hard work and dedication to rehabilitating my knee and learning as much as I could would get me there. I used that fuel to help myself gain strength, lose body fat, and most importantly, gain confidence inside and outside of the gym. I graduated college with a total count of one knee surgery, some amazing experience working with NCAA athletes and personal training clients alike, and one degree in Kinesiology. I did it!

I moved to Nashville, Tennessee after graduating and starting working at Vanderbilt Orthopedic Institute teaching boot camp classes, conducting post rehabilitation training sessions alongside the physical therapy staff, and conducting functional movement screens for members of the facility. I gained so much experience working in this environment but something was missing. Nashville felt small to me and I was homesick for Atlanta so I quickly changed plans, moved back to Atlanta and started working in gym sales and management in order to gain experience in areas I wasn't comfortable with.

Luckily, I learned many lessons despite struggling for money and not earning many commissions dollars because I wasn't a hot shot sales woman. My focus was leadership among the staff of personal trainers and I made many relationships at that facility that are still with me now. Today, I am still personal training but I have gone to great lengths to try and gain as much extra education as possible on my mission of changing the world of knees. I work at an incredible personal training studio that allows me to use my knowledge every day to help others decrease pain and cure nagging injuries in their lives. My goal is to get my Master's degree in Biomechanics and Doctorate in Physical Therapy which will further promote my mission of being the ACL expert. Terry and I met for lunch to catch up on old times and more importantly talk about Tennessee football. During our conversation, he asked how my knees were doing and I responded by telling him that I was constantly in pain but worked on corrective exercise, mobility techniques, and gaining strength on a daily and weekly basis to ensure the best pain relief, safety, and longevity for my knees. Terry told me that the amount of pain I was experiencing was not normal and he wanted to look at my knee. He concluded that my left ACL was not functional.

I thought it was a joke. There was no way this could be happening to me again. There was no way I was going through this again. He must be joking, right? It was worse than he thought. After meeting with two different surgeons I finally received the answers I needed and realized because of how much my knees had been through I had to seek out the best surgeon in Atlanta. Dr. Tom Myers and his highly renowned double- bundled ACL surgery seemed to be the only procedure that would work on someone like me who has had multiple revision surgeries on each knee leaving my knees even looser than before. I also learned with each ACL surgery I had in the past, the surgeons had to drill a tunnel in my lower leg and a tunnel in my upper leg in order to securely screw the new ACL in place. Essentially, I had two separate tunnels in my left knee and they were way too big to support another ACL surgery or another tunnel. In fact, I was starting to run the risk of having a knee fracture because the hole in my bone was more than twice the size it should have been.

The ACL used in my last ACL surgery in high school was a cadaver graft and the cadaver in my left knee had slowly failed over time and had started to disintegrate inside of my knee. Apparently, cadaver grafts have a much higher failure rate; I was not told these risks by my second surgeon in high school. Now, because of the overly large tunnels in my knee, I needed two surgeries to fix the problem: One surgery to remove the faulty ACL and add in bone chips to heal over a period of six months, and a subsequent surgery to fix the ACL and possibly the ALL. I never re-injured myself but because my cadaver ACL slowly failed over time, I also tore my MCL and meniscus just through the general wear and tear of not having a functional ACL to stabilize my knee. Even worse, we had no way to see if the cadaver in my right knee was going to stay in tract or not. What if I had to face two more surgeries on both knees? How was I possibly going to afford these out-of-pocket expenses and keep up my non-contact personal training job on my feet all day? How was I going to afford my Masters and Doctorate degrees now? Am I strong enough to go through all of this again, and again?

I cannot answer these questions and I have learned that worrying about the answers to these questions only makes me lose a moment of happiness right now. I had my bone graft and ACL removal surgery on my 27th birthday. My plans to attend a Master's Degree program were put on hold in order to prioritize rehabilitation and recovery. My focus for the next six months while awaiting ACL surgery was to gain as much strength as possible in order to ensure that my recovery from ACL surgery would be a smoother process. I began writing down positive affirmations every single day to keep my mind focused on the present day and what I could control in order to avoid being scared and overwhelmed. Little did I know these affirmations would give me the courage and confidence to change my life. I had started a book on ACL Injury Prevention a few months prior, but kept hitting roadblocks with my set up and structure. All of a sudden I sat down and just began writing everything I was knew about the approach and recovery from ACL surgery. I knew other athletes could benefit from my experiences and the plethora of information I had been studying and researching since I was 13-years-old. Upon my own amazement, within only three short months, I had finished almost an entire book and had developed my own website. The fuel inside of me was sparked by my recent diagnosis and it was time to make things happen instead of waiting for them to come to me. There are too many other athletes out there suffering similar situations as I am and they deserve a change and a tool to use for their recoveries.

Unfortunately, my recovery wasn't going exactly as planned. I lived on the 4th floor with no access to an elevator and the very severe degree of instability in my knee caused by the fact that I had no ACL, and a torn meniscus and MCL, made the stairs grueling and agonizing. My schedule at work training clients was also causing me increased levels of pain. Being on my feet ten hours per day wasn't easy on this knee with no ACL, and my other knee, which has had multiple surgeries too, was taking the brunt of the load and becoming very painful as well.

It is interesting going on a journey like this because while many other athletes have unfortunately needed multiple revision surgeries like I have, most of these athletes are also going through these surgeries at similar time frames as me. We are essentially the first round of athletes to require so many procedures. My surgeon, athletic trainer, and I have had to realize this is not something where we have proven recovery methods and scholarly articles to read to affirm our tactics and my potential outcome. I am one of few athletes requiring this many revisions and while it is becoming more common, we are the athletes paving the way for the next generation of athletes. We are sacrificing our knees for change. We will be the future outcome studies for the experts to analyze and evaluate.

We don't know with certainty the condition our knees will be in later in life. But we do know that the quality of life now without functioning ACL grafts is not allowing us for the active lifestyle we desire. It is my mission to change these statistics and situations for the next generation of athletes and it must start now. We need to create increased awareness for ACL injuries and ACL injury prevention now. We need to start performing better ACL reconstructions now. We need to make up for the lack of insurance visits for rehabilitation now. When you tear your ACL, your life is changed forever. I never thought I'd be facing a 7th surgery. I didn't think it was physically possible and my 13-year-old self would be disgusted with what has happened to me. But it took until my most recent and hopefully last ACL journey to truly realize the lesson I needed to learn. Surviving 7 has changed my life and Surviving 7 will help me change the lives of many athletes for years to come.

Surviving 7 means despite the obstacles standing in my way, I can create change in the world of knees and in the way we approach ACL injury and surgery. It means I will prevent others from suffering the same fate and it means I will recover from number 7 for the ACL family. Surviving 7 is for every single person who has torn their ACL and knows what it means for the quickest instant to change your athletic career forever. Surviving 7 will help me to inspire anyone struggling with their ACL recovery; that they too are strong enough mentally and physically to beat the odds and they need to approach their recovery with the utmost importance in order to prevent re-injury and regression from their sport. *Surviving 7* will help me deliver my message to the world so everyone will learn and understand the increased risk for female athletes, ages 12-17, and create change in the industry to prevent young girls from dealing with season ending surgeries and a lifetime of struggle with their knees.

Surviving 7 is for the future athletes who will tear their ACL and will need a guide to a functional and exceptional recovery in order to decrease their risk of subsequent ACL tear. Surviving 7 is for all the moms and dads who watched their young daughters be strong and persevere through a surgery that Adrian Peterson made popular. *Surviving 7* is meant to change the way we approach ACL surgery and to raise the standard for the quality of care of our youth athletes. Surviving 7 is meant to light a fire under the rears of the surgeons who try to fit in as many surgeries per day as they can with fast cadaver procedures without being honest about the risks to their patients.

Surviving 7 is meant to raise awareness to ACL injury and the fact that quality ACL Injury Prevention Programs should be available in all cities for any youth sports teams. Surviving 7 is meant to raise awareness on the risk of re-injury; after tearing your ACL one time, you have a 1 in 50 chance of tearing it again. Surviving 7 is meant to tell the world that while the female athlete has MANY anatomical, structural, hormonal, and environmental factors against them, together we can decrease ACL injury rates in women and prepare our female athletes to dominate in every aspect of life. This book is meant to change the world of knees!

Please use this book as a guide to learning how your ACL injury happened, how to prevent subsequent ACL injury, and how to get through this surgery mentally and physically from a 7-time knee surgery survivor (5 total ACL.) Each surgery has presented different challenges for me and sharing all my tips will help you to avoid some of the problems I have encountered so that you can have a smoother recovery and hopefully never need a revision surgery. Learn as much as you can about the knee and how your body mechanics can increase or decrease your risk of ACL injury. The more well-known these risks become the easier it will be to implement ACL injury prevention programs around the country. I hope this inspires you and helps you to confront this journey with courage and hope. Enjoy.

2

KNEE BACKGROUND

THE KNEE

E veryone scrapes it, bumps it, and bruises it, but what is really going on in there? It is a relatively simple joint when you compare it to others in the body. It is exposed to forces that can exceed five times the weight of the body. But, it has enhanced mobility at the cost of stability. This is important because our knees are able to bend and extended to great range of motion put these capabilities also it at increased risk for injury. An unstable knee will usually cause pain and weakness resulting in an injury at some point. Decreased stability at the knee is a major source of pain and injury for many people. It can be said that those with decreased stability at the knee have a higher chance of tearing their ACL. Learning more about the complexity of the knee joint can help us to fix issues in the lower body to aid the performance and increase stability at the knee joint, in turn decreasing the risk of ACL injury.

The knee is a basic hinge joint which means it mostly works in flexion and extension (bend and straighten) movements and has very little medial or lateral rotation (side-to-side rotation.) Think of your knee like a door hinge. The hinge itself is very secure and screwed into place but it is also connected to the wall and the door. If the wall or the door becomes unstable then the hinge not only becomes unstable, too, but has to bear the extra load in order to open and close the door. This is similar to the relationship between your foot/ankle, knee, and hip. Your knee is the hinge and the foot/ankle and hip are the wall and door. The hinge will only be as strong and functional as its support system and all of those moving parts work together to build a sound and supportive door. The body is a kinetic chain, meaning all the parts are connected and a dysfunction in any piece of the chain can cause problems on either end. Dysfunctions and different angles of the feet and hips put the knee joint at risk of harm in numerous ways. It is the joint stuck in the middle of two very complicated joints that have extremely common dysfunctions making the knee increasingly prone to pain and injury.

The knee is the largest joint in the body and one of the most easily injured. It is made up of four main things: ligaments, tendons, bone, and cartilage. The knee comes together with the bottom of the femur (thigh bone) and the top of the tibia (lower leg bone). The patella tendon connects the kneecap (patella) to the shinbone (tibia) and is attached to the quadriceps muscles by the quadriceps tendon. The quadriceps muscles, quadriceps tendon, and patella tendon work together to straighten the knee. The main ligaments of the knee are the ACL, PCL, MCL, and LCL. Essentially the ACL and PCL, located in the center of the knee, work together to stabilize the knee and protect it from sliding in front of the tibia, hyperextending, and having too much rotation. The MCL is in the inner side of the knee and the LCL is on the outside of the knee. These ligaments work to control the side to side stability of the knee joint. The meniscus is a rubbery C-shaped disc that cushions your knee, and each knee has two menisci one on the inner edge and one on the outer edge. The menisci help to keep your knee steady by balancing your weight across the knee.

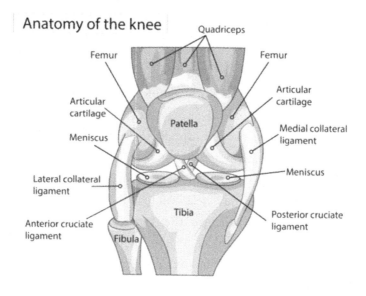

Like most joints in the body, the knee is a synovial joint. Synovial joints get lubrication to aid and enhance their movements from synovial fluid. It's kind of like using a lubricant on a rusty gear or machine part. Synovial fluid is naturally produced and excreted in the body through movement. Do you know the feeling of stiffness and pain you get after sitting for a prolonged period of time? This is due to many factors, but one of them is the decrease in production of synovial fluid. The body is extremely efficient and has come up with its own pain reliever, but the body is smart and will not produce the synovial fluid unless you are moving. Because logically speaking, if you aren't moving around then you won't be in pain, right? Not really, but the body will not waste energy on producing synovial fluid unless it thinks you need it and when you are sedentary the body stops producing it. The next time you are stiff and complain of knee pain it might be better to go on a walk or ride a bike for 15 minutes in order to get yourself moving, blood flowing, and synovial fluid production increase.

While the knee can be fairly simple in comparison to the hip, shoulder, or ankle it also heavily relies on its major functioning ligaments for support. Injury to any of these ligaments can create major problems for an active person or an athlete. Most everyone has had knee pain or a knee injury before. Everyday wear and tear and overuse injuries are very common because the knee is a sitting duck between the hip and ankle. When there are compromised movements or range of motion restrictions at the hip or ankle, the knee is the joint that has to take over and sometimes not in a good way. But sudden or acute injuries are the most common cause of knee problems. Sports like soccer, basketball, football, and volleyball have a high incidence of knee injuries but even twisting wrong or taking a wrong step can also cause an acute knee injury.

This shows how faulty mechanics and improper movement patterns can easily lead to a knee injury and by learning more about the biomechanics of the lower body it is possible to decrease the risk of injury and pain at your knee.

2.2 WHAT IS THE ACL?

The ACL or Anterior Cruciate Ligament is the main ligament in the front or anterior portion of the knee that assists in deceleration movements and changing directions. It consists of two fiber bundles; the anteromedial and the posterolateral bundle. When the knee is extended or straightened the posterolateral bundle is tight and the anteromedial bundle is slightly lax. Conversely when the knee is flexed or bent, the anteromedial bundle tightens and the posterolateral bundle relaxes. This anatomical double bundle ACL is important to note when we talk about ACL reconstruction in Chapter 5. The ACL prevents the tibia from sliding out in front of the femur and creates rotational stability for the knee joint. The ACL works in conjunction with the PCL or Posterior Cruciate Ligament which is located on the posterior side of the knee and prevents the tibia from moving backwards too far (or hyperextending). The PCL is less common to injure because it normally happens from a tackle to the front of the knees or hyperextension at the knee.

It's kind of like the ACL is a little rubber band inside of your knee holding your knee in place between your lower leg and your upper leg. If that rubber band were to become too stretched out or even partially torn or fully torn, then your knee will start to flop around forward and backward, and rotate too much. While it is possible to lead a functional life with this loosened or ripped rubber band, you can see how it will make easy tasks very hard to do and simple things like walking up and down the stairs painful. Conversely, ACL tears are the most common knee injury and athletes participating in sports such as soccer, football, basketball, and volleyball have an increased chance of injury because of the high demand of cutting, acceleration, deceleration, jumping and landing, and contact qualities of the sports. ACL injuries occur in more than 200,000 cases in the United States each year and extensive surgical and rehabilitative costs exceed $650 million annually in the American Health Care system[2].

Close to 70% of ACL injuries are non-contact in nature; meaning they happen during a bad landing from a jump or when an athlete changes direction. The non-contact ACL injuries typically happen because of a structural issue in the kinetic chain[3]. Remember, everything in the body is connected and one dysfunction can cause dysfunction above and below the problem. Now remember the door hinge example? Your foot is the wall, your knee is the hinge, and your hip is the door. The wall has a foundation problem and begins to get weaker over time causing the door to lean a little bit. The hinge is unable to support these new structural changes and instead attempts to maintain support by using the screws as its main support system instead of the entire system together. Eventually with one quick opening of the door, the screw (ACL) breaks and the hinge has no support left.

Because of our chair bound lifestyles humans have more

dysfunctions in their bodies now than ever before! Just like the foundation problem at the wall, we can pinpoint and fix biomechanical compensations in your body. You are what you repeatedly do, and your body molds to the chair you sit in all day. When you step onto the volleyball court or go to the gym to do a squat, your body is going to mimic and replicate the positions it is used to; meaning your improper form is going to translate into your muscle memory and into the motions you perform every day. Your ankles are tight and your hips are weak from sitting all day. Now, you are landing from an amazing layup in a pickup basketball game with your friends and all of a sudden your leg buckles and you feel a pop. That's all it takes.

One reason the ACL is so susceptible to injury is because it is a major feedback spot in the knee. When the support systems of the foot and hip above and below the knee have dysfunction, it is the knee's job to continue on as normal. But the knee doesn't have as many intricate tendons or intrinsic receptor muscles like the foot and hip do. The foundation of everything you do starts with your foot and your foot is wired directly to the pelvic floor muscles in the core to let the body know where it is in space and how to control it. Because the knee is so simple, it doesn't have all of that but it does have the ACL. The ACL is a mechanoreceptor. Mechanoreceptors provide information to the Central Nervous System regarding touch, pressure, position, or distortion; basically, allowing the body to know where it is in space and react to different stimuli. ACL mechanoreceptors are a crucial part of the proprioceptive sensitivity of the knee and contribute to functional stability at the knee joint. Essentially, the ACL provides your brain with feedback about positions and movements in real speed time as they are happening. Injury to the ACL can be detrimental because it causes damage to these mechanoreceptors (or space awareness sensors) triggering mechanical instability and a disturbance to the neuromuscular control of the injured knee. This basically means that after suffering an ACL injury it is common to experience decreased response and control of that knee, as well as instability that causes knee pain. This actually makes the athlete even more prone to re-injury because one side of the body will have deviations from the other following an ACL injury.

Recent studies show that although damage to the ACL can play a significant role on proprioceptive (or knowing where you are in space) potential of the knee, autograft surgeries can help to restore mechanoreceptors of the ACL but results vary based on duration of injury and other interdependent factors. This means that after injury to the ACL it can be very hard for an athlete to restore their normal reaction times and relearn their proprioceptive ability or the awareness of their knee in positions and movements. Sometimes this is thought of as a mental block or being scared to perform certain movements again following an injury but it has just as much to do with the decreased neuromuscular awareness stemming from the damaged or missing mechanoreceptors as it does the brain itself. This can play a huge role in the risk of re-injuring your ACL because a decrease in proprioceptive abilities of the knee can contribute to improper cutting, jumping, or landing mechanics further contributing to your risk of ACL tear. Remember, about 70-75% or ¾ of ACL injuries are non-contact injuries but with proper strength training programs and coaches working with athletes on jumping, landing, and cutting movements a lot of these injuries and re-injures can be prevented[3].

All of the contributing factors effecting ACL tear incidence in athletes are staggering but the worst part is after suffering an ACL injury on one knee the athlete goes from a 1 and 3,500 chance of sustaining an ACL injury (although the incidence rate might actually be higher) to a 1 in 50 chance either on the repaired graft or on the uninjured knee. This is a huge difference and every athlete with previous ACL injury should be aware of these risks so that a proper injury prevention program can be put in place[2]. My mission is to raise awareness to these staggering statistics and ensure that all athletes who tear their ACL find a quality injury prevention program to help them change their injury risk as well as implement ACL injury prevention training programs to all youth female athletic teams because of their higher incidence rates.

3

THE KNEE, THERE IS A DIFFERENCE BETWEEN MEN AND WOMEN

WOMEN AND THE ACL

Many of us are aware of the increased risk of ACL injury in female athletes but how bad is it really? Studies show that female athletes are 2-8 times more likely to tear their ACL than their male counterparts[3]. There are many factors contributing to these statistics but the good news is there are ways to prevent ACL injuries and screening methods to expose athletes that are more at risk. By understanding the risk factors and the different anatomical and biomechanical aspects contributing to ACL injury risk in the female athlete, we can better prepare our female athletes for long term success in their sport of choice. Coaches, parents, and female athletes alike should have a basic understanding of why young female athletes do have an increased risk of ACL injury and the more people that learn these principles the more likely it will be to begin to implement simple prevention programs into team warm ups and conditioning drills.

The issues contributing to ACL injury risk in women range in variation from environmental, structural, hormonal, anatomical, and muscular based; but while we cannot change every single aspect; when addressed, many contributing factors can dramatically decrease the prevalence of ACL injury risk. By interpreting the different biomechanical deviations of athletes and using corrective exercise and strength training programs to fix abnormalities contributing to extra stress and force on the knee joint, the risk of ACL tear decreases substantially.

Female athletes are more at risk for an ACL tear during the ages of 12 to 17 because their bodies are changing. There are increased levels of hormones, primarily a large increase in estrogen, and the pelvis begins to widen causing new geometrical angles for the athlete's body to learn to adapt to. But just like you need to break in a new pair of shoes before you go running in them, we need to realize that our young female athletes need to train and prepare their new bodies to play sports. The different geometrical angles at the hips and knees require a solid foundation of core strength, stabilization strength, and corrective exercise for weakened muscles in order to prevent injury. Without proper training, these young athletes cannot possibly keep up with how fast their body is changing and it's only a matter of time before their soccer game ends with a nasty injury. The female body wasn't designed for sports like the male body, but we can change the significance of the design flaws regarding sport and performance which will better prepare female athletes for success without injury.

ACL surgery has detrimental long-term effects on anyone. It is a major procedure and any type of surgery is going to cause pain and increase the prevalence for re-injury, and arthritis long term. The fact that hundreds of thousands of young teenage girls are facing these surgeries head on needs to resonate with our industry into causing a revelation of change. Children should not have to carry physical trauma into adulthood. The adult body comes with enough pain and injuries just through our lifestyles and the aging process so it is scary to think what all of the ACL comeback stories will turn out to be when these children are 60 and 80. We do not have many long-term studies on these repercussions because before sports were popular among women we were not aware of the increased prevalence of ACL tear for youth female athletes. It is devastating to know that simple changes in training methods can decrease such a damaging injury but in many circumstances, no one is aware of their increased risk or even aware of the small measures that could be implemented to create positive change. Now that we are aware of the risks, it is time to use our knowledge to create change for the next generation of young female athletes.

3.1.1 STRUCTURAL AND ANATOMICAL RISK

The increased risk of ACL injury in female athletes is due to multiple factors including differences in structure like the size of the knee. The size and shape of the knee joint is typically much smaller in women than in men due to the overall size difference of a woman versus a man. Smaller size of the knee causes the ACL to get caught and tear more easily than a larger size. Picture the structure of a woman's knee looking like the shape of the letter V and the structure of a man's looking like the letter U. The ACL in the V knee has much less space and will much more likely get caught and tear versus the ACL in the U has ample room to glide as the femur and tibia translate into knee flexion and extension.

Some of these differences in size relate to the tibial plateau. The tibial plateau is a spot in the knee where the tibia (lower leg) helps to form the actual knee joint. Think of it as the top portion of your lower leg bone that is underneath your knee cap forming the bottom part of the knee joint. It is one of the most important weight bearing areas in the human body. The increase in slope in the V knee causes an increase in anterior translation of the knee basically meaning that those people with an increased slope in the tibial plateau also have an increase in force on the front of the knee in rotation and twisting motions. One of the main mechanisms of the ACL is to prevent anterior translation at the knee and it is very common for an ACL to completely rupture due to excessive anterior translation. That being said, those with an increase in slope at the tibial plateau like most females and some males tend to have a much larger incidence for ACL injury because of the increase in force at the spot in the knee.

Differences in hip width cause an increased Q angle in most women compared to men. The Q angle is the angle measuring from midpoint of the patella (kneecap) to the ASIS at the hip. The larger the angle the greater the lateral force on the patella or kneecap, creating more force at the knee. The increased force on the knees stemming from the larger Q angle puts the knee in more compromised positions more often than that of a smaller Q angle causing many more situations to occur that could result in a possible ACL tear. Because the teenage female athlete is going through maturation changes that widen her hips, she quickly becomes more prone to ACL tear.

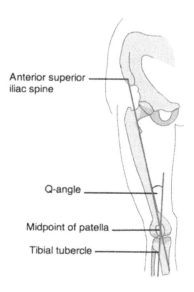

A normal Q angle in women is about 17-degrees and a normal Q angle in men is 14-degrees. While only a 3-degree difference doesn't sound like very much, picture every step you take and every time you walk up and down stairs your knee just has slightly more force on it than it should. Overtime this will add up and most likely cause wear and tear and painful symptoms to occur. Pain is a late indicator of a problem so by this time your body has naturally compensated to prevent this pain for a long time and most likely has thrown off the way your leg muscles should be firing and working in order to keep your pain level down. While this is efficient and helpful to manage pain, it is not helpful when it comes to your risk of injury as certain muscles are working inadequately, which will increase your risk of injury. Also, remember that 14-degrees for men and 17-degrees for women is normal but anything higher than normal increases lateral force to the knee substantially. Many women have Q angles that measure much wider than 17-degrees.

Because these angles are the anatomy we are born with or develop as a result of puberty, it is impossible to change your Q angle but it is highly recommended to learn how your Q angle affects your risk of injury. By incorporating an effective strength training and rehabilitation program, altering the biomechanics will help to decrease pain and injury risk associated with the Q angle. Strong and dominant muscles need to be stretched and relaxed so that the weaker muscles can be strengthened and help to re-alter the mechanics of your knee. In most cases the VMO muscle or the Vastus Mediailis Oblique (a part of the quads located directly above the knee to the inside) is weak and those fibers play an important role in the stability and positioning of the patella (knee cap). Another common weak muscle is the Gluteus Medius (a small abductor muscle in the glutes) and with strengthening methods could help to decrease force on the knee resulting from a larger Q angle. By restoring strength and firing sequences to this muscle and increasing strength at the hips, the impact of a larger Q angle will have less affect. "The absence of increased hip abduction strength in adolescent girls as they mature may be related to their emergent increased risk of ACL during adolescence. These findings may indicate that strength and conditioning protocols that include hip abduction strengthening should be implemented for young girls beginning at age 12 to 13, when the divergence between girls and boys begin to occur."[4]

Another common occurrence in female athletes is over pronation at the foot. Over pronation is when the foot naturally rolls inwards during a walking or running motion. Pronation at the foot is natural to help the body to absorb shock but over pronation is a problem which can cause issues with the arch at your foot and issues up the entire kinetic chain. In regards to the knee, over pronation at the foot forces the knee to internally rotate producing more stress with each motion. Remember the body is a kinetic chain, if your foot rolls inward during every step you take then so is your knee, creating shear forces on the knee joint that could possibly wear out at any time. Athletes with larger Q angles and an over pronating foot have many more compromised positions for the knees even in a normal walking gait. This can mean potential chronic trauma to many of the structures in the knee; cartilage, ligaments, tendons. The body naturally adapts to these movement patterns and when this same athlete plays basketball or soccer they are significantly more likely to tear their ACL just because of the mechanisms of how their body moves.

Over pronation at the foot can be caused by either foot instability or hip instability. Over pronation at the foot is much more common in females because women typically have weaker hips than men. The major culprit muscle is a weak or under activated gluteus medius muscle which is a stabilizing muscle on the sides of the butt. Having a weak gluteus medius can cause the leg to roll inwards during every step.

At the time of heel strike during the walking or running gait pattern, the knee is usually fully extended or has about 20-degrees of flexion (bend), and the forces transmitted from the foot to the knee are very high. When extension or slight flexion is combined with internal rotation at the lower leg (stemming from over pronation at the foot) it is an extremely common position for ACL tears. For an athlete with normal foot pronation it is much easier to recover from this vulnerable position quickly and easily. But for the athlete with excessive over pronation at the foot, this position is going to be more over pronounced and harder to quickly recover from. The foot rolls inward more in the athlete with the over pronation problem which produces excessive force up the kinetic chain into the knee. This causes improper force vector at the quadriceps and overtime can cause tracking issues at the knee cap creating more stress on the inside or medial side of the knee. The increased risk of ACL injury for this over pronated foot athlete happens every time they play sports. Eventually the shear forces on the knee in this single leg position described above give out and an ACL tear occurs.

The body's first contact to the ground starts with the foot. By addressing over pronation problems in the foot and strengthening the gluteus medius in the hips and stabilizers in the foot to correct the over pronation problem it is easy to decrease foot pronation and allow the athlete to perform with less strain and pain to the knee and decreased risk of ACL injury.

Now imagine you are an avid runner suffering from over pronation at the foot. Every run you go on is increasing the wear on your knee. You decide to play a game of sand volleyball on your next beach vacation and your body is so programmed to continue rolling the foot and knee inward, when you take a wrong step in the sand you instantly tear your ACL. This is how easy it can happen! Proper corrective exercise techniques could have been applied to improve your foot pronation and increase your gluteus medius strength, reducing the wear on your knee during your runs and decreasing your risk of tearing your ACL.

Similar to over pronation at the foot, Knee Valgus is a common trait of many female athletes. Knee valgus is when the knee naturally buckles inward during a load like a squat. Knee valgus is very common in men and women alike but because of the larger Q angle in women and increased over pronation of the foot in some women; knee valgus can be a lot more detrimental to a female athlete than a male. Women are much more prone to having knee valgus because of weak hips, wider Q angle, and being taught to sit like a lady for all of their life. Repeated positions like sitting with the legs crossed can cause further muscle compensations leading to increased knee valgus over time. Most knee valgus in male and females occurs because of weak hips, tight ankles, and impaired quad and hamstring function. Again, these are all common dysfunctions that occur from sitting too much.

Athletes with valgus knee tendencies are much more likely to suffer from knee pain and eventually a knee injury because of the increase in force at the knee joint. It is no coincidence that similar tight and weak muscle groups cause knee valgus and over pronation at the foot. Combine this valgus knee tendency with a wide Q angle and an over pronated foot and you have a recipe for disaster. Think of it this way, the ACL, unfortunately, is able to loosen and unwind with certain movements. Remember from the knee joint overview in section 1.1, the ACL works in conjunction with the PCL. They are cruciate ligaments which means they cross each other almost like you would cross your fingers. During movements that turn the knees inward like someone squatting with knee valgus; this motion actually unwinds the ACL causing it to loosen and weaken. But movements where the knees safely turn out a little wind the ACL up and are much safer to perform. Repetitive motions of knee valgus can contribute to loosening at the ACL because of the unwinding tendency of that motion to the ACL. It is obvious then, the best focus for squatting is to have the knees turn out slightly. This will reinforce safe movement patterns that will translate onto the playing field. Similar to the Q angle and an overly pronated foot, knee valgus can be addressed with a proper rehabilitation program which can help to considerably decrease pain and injury risk associated with these anatomical variations. Addressing the tight ankles and increasing strength in the hips, glutes, quads, and hamstrings can significantly reduce knee valgus tendencies.

3.1.2 NEUROMUSCULAR IMBALANCES

It's not a secret, men and women are created differently. Men have increased levels of testosterone which helps them to build and maintain more muscle mass than women. This can play an impact in the competitive female athlete because she is automatically more predisposed to having weaknesses that will contribute to pain and injury. A decrease in neuromuscular control is common in women and puts passive stress on the ligaments in the knee. Neuromuscular control is basically the connection between the brain and muscles telling which muscles to fire and when, and the muscles, tendons, and ligaments providing feedback to the brain. A decrease in neuromuscular control makes an athlete more vulnerable because improper firing sequencing in muscles lead to compensations in movement which make you more prone to chronic stress and injury.

Women are also more likely to have leg dominance issues. Leg dominance occurs typically when the dominant leg is stronger than the non-dominant leg. Most athletes have a dominant leg that they kick, throw, or shoot with but female athletes are more likely to have a difference in strength from the dominant leg to the non-dominant leg. Any time there are discrepancies on one side of the body versus the other, the athlete is more prone to injury because of the change in efficiency of the mechanics involved in certain motions preformed. This can happen when one leg is stronger than the other, when one leg is more flexible or mobile than the other, or as discussed previously; when an injury results in decreased reaction time on one side versus the other. In either case, there are differences from one side to the other making that athlete more vulnerable because the body will have to generate compensations in order to continue to produce efficient movements.

This is important to note because any athlete who has had a previous injury and especially any athlete who has had an ACL surgery is going to be more prone to experiencing leg dominance. Leg dominance is one of the main reasons that ACL injury incidence rates increase after having one ACL injury. After tearing your ACL you have a 1 in 50 chance of tearing it again or tearing the ACL in the other knee. Because of these issues it is very important to successfully complete an entire rehabilitation and strength training program before advancing to running, cutting, and jumping drills. If there is even the slightest difference in strength or flexibility in one leg versus the other your chances of injury increase.

Soccer in particular is a sport where many athletes experience ACL tears. It is interesting because soccer athletes are more likely to have asymmetries in one leg versus the other due to the nature of the sport; planting and kicking the ball with the same dominant leg hundreds and hundreds of times. It is interesting to note that studies have concluded that male soccer players are more likely to injure the ACL on their dominant or kicking leg while female soccer players are more likely to injure the ACL on the non-dominant or planting leg. This speaks volumes to the fact the because of the weaker hip and hamstring muscles in female athletes the non-contact planting leg is much more vulnerable to ACL injury.[5]

Neuromuscular training programs help to eliminate this issue and are specifically important for the female athlete to incorporate and master because female athletes typically have altered firing patterns in their muscles unlike most males. Neuromuscular training programs are crucial for any athlete recovering from or preventing ACL injury.

On top of having a general decrease in muscle mass compared to men, most females are quad dominant meaning they heavily utilize the quadriceps muscles during actions that require quads, hamstrings, and glutes. This is important to note because if the muscles are not firing in the proper sequencing there could be a delay in the firing sequence causing the athlete to be more prone to injury. For example, the hamstrings control eccentric forces and help an athlete to safely slow down after accelerating. If there is a delay in the firing of the hamstring complex (where the quads fire first) then that muscle group is not able to fire quickly enough to help the athlete safely decelerate causing the ACL to take over and ultimately sprain or tear. It is ideal is for the hamstring complex to be at least 60% of quadriceps strength. In addition to messing up the proper firing sequencing, quad dominance also creates increased wear on the knee joint over time particularly at the Patella Tendon (kneecap) because it is attached to the quadriceps complex via the quadriceps tendon. If the athlete has strong hamstrings and glutes those muscles will work together to load the forces of the movements of the body more to the posterior chain or muscles on the back side of the body. This is important because it takes pressure off the knees and the lower back.

On top of the decreased firing sequences of the hamstring complex, many women have trouble building up their VMO muscle in the quadriceps. This will sound strange given that most women are quad dominant but because of the wider Q angle the VMO muscle receives less stress. The VMO or Vastus Mediailis Oblique, is one of the four quadriceps muscles located toward the inner part of your thigh. It is normally very well developed even in an out of shape male but in women it is often under pronounced and not as functional. When underdeveloped the muscle can cause tracking issues in the Patella or knee cap which can relate to the pain associated with Runner's Knee. Atrophy in a single muscle in the quadriceps can cause major dysfunction to the lower body. This is important to note when talking about ACL injury because by strengthening this muscle, it will help to maintain normal function at the knee which is always a priority when trying to decrease pain and injury.

Anytime there are muscle imbalances the athlete has an increased injury risk. But this is not a limiting factor! Strength training benefits for both genders are incredible and an increase in knowledge and available strength training programs for young female athletes is a huge way to not only provide them with a healthy foundation and approach to maintaining strength throughout their lives but will also decrease many injury risks that come from having muscle weakness. Comprehensive neuromuscular training programs can help the female athlete to decrease gender related differences increasing their injury risk and also increasing strength, power, and neuromuscular control. It is perfectly okay for our youth to participate in weekly resistance training workouts even if their bodies are growing and changing. They sit at school all day long; so without a proper resistance training program children in America today already have major dysfunctions from being desk bound. Athletes need resistance training to prepare their bodies for sport and grow stronger.

3.1.3 INFLUENCE OF HORMONES

The hormones associated with puberty in females provide the foundation for the body to develop and change from a child to that of a woman. Estrogen levels increase, a menstrual cycle begins, and the pelvis widens to support the birthing process and child bearing capabilities one day. That is a whole lot going on in a 12 to 17-year-old girl! All of that change is new for the body and it can have many diverse side effects associated with different levels of estrogen. No matter what, that much change in any body is enough to disrupt the system. Take that disrupted system, without preventative training to account for new hormones and new angles at the pelvis, and throw it onto a soccer field, and you can see how increased risks associated with puberty in a woman can be very disadvantageous for an athlete.

But even more alarming than the physiological changes during puberty affecting athletes, research shows estrogen has effects on the ACL. Estrogen is known to play a role in the structure of the ACL. The hormones in the menstrual cycle influence ACL tear rate by altering the structure of the ACL. These hormones, specifically estrogen, bind to the ACL decreasing the tensile integrity and collagen production of the ACL. The ACL and many other ligaments in the body are comprised of high levels of collagen in order to maintain their structure. This could theoretically increase injury incidence rates of ACL tears during the pre-ovulatory phase spanning 1 to 14 days of the menstrual cycle where estrogen is more prominent. Because higher estrogen levels are typically recorded in women during puberty and childbearing age there is a much higher incidence of ACL tear in women of those ages, specifically during the teenage years. Although all of the hormones involved in a normal functioning menstrual cycle are the same, there are varying levels of hormones for each woman and for each time frame of life. This means some women will have more effects of estrogen on the ACL than others all based on hormone levels.

The hormones associated with a woman's menstrual cycle also put women at an increased risk of injury because at a certain phase during the monthly cycle all of the ligaments in a women's body get very lax. This prepares the body for childbirth one day. Imagine stepping onto the soccer field with all of your ligaments in a laxity phase. It would be like all of your joints are made of Gumby material; a recipe for disaster.

Now I'm certainly not advocating that all women should stop playing sports during the 1 to 14 days where there is increased estrogen production in the menstrual cycle but with all of these factors contributing to the high incidence of ACL tears in female athletes it further concludes to the fact that ACL Injury Prevention Programs should be in place for all competitive female athletic teams starting from age 10-12. With sedentary lifestyles and high fat diets, young girls are going through puberty at earlier ages so this age range could potentially start even younger as well. The bottom line is know your risks so you can change your results. Prepare your young athletes for the demands of their sports and they will hopefully not have to face season ending injuries resulting in high medical bills, grueling rehabilitation, increased risk of re injury, and increased risk of developing arthritis.

3.1.4 ENVIRONMENTAL EFFECTS

Because of all of these forces working against a female athletes' knee, it is essential to include prevention based strength training methods and proper plyometric training programs to ensure the athlete is prepared for cutting, decelerating, and landing properly. Almost 70% of ACL injuries occur in a non-contact manor so the effectiveness of these strength training programs on reducing ACL injuries could be immense! But not all women's athletic teams have an educated and dedicated strength staff, especially at the youth level where girls are increasingly at risk.

Many male youth sports teams have hired a knowledgeable staff for pre and post-season training. This is not always the case for female sports teams due to lack of funding and lack of interest. Men's teams usually have a larger following creating the increase in funding but for female athletics team it's important to get creative in order to raise money to hire adequate strength training and injury prevention specialists. At the youth level it is uncommon to do any type of strength training or change of direction drills, but remember, the female athletes are most at risk of ACL tear during the ages of 12 to 17 so this creates a big hole in the system. The athletes who are statistically the most prone for injury are receiving little to no help to prevent those measures.

The culture of women's athletics needs to change in order for women and their coaches to take themselves and their preparation for sport seriously. In men's athletics there are no excuses, you either work hard, train, and prepare; or you don't play. I have watched girls on my previous teams lie to get out of running or whine and complain the coach was working them too hard. This simply does not exist in male sports. These small environmental changes can end up causing an injury long term because if you are not prepared for your sport then your body will suffer. It's time for female athletes to have the confidence and courage to ask for more help and demand more respect for their competition and preparation for competition. If you are a female athlete don't fret! This isn't supposed to scare you it is supposed to motivate you to seek knowledge and a comprehensive training program so we can change the ACL incidence injury rate.

Make sure your daughter's youth sports programs have adequate strength training and plyometric training programs in place. They are not too young to start a training program, especially if they are playing the sport competitively. If they do not have a certified professional, then it is okay to seek one out. Try searching on Google or LinkedIn for a Strength and Conditioning Specialist, Personal Trainer, or Athletic Trainer with Injury Prevention Specializations. You could contract this employ to do workshops with your sports teams or even do individual screenings on athletes to find the ones with increased injury risk. Many times, simply incorporating a progressive based strength training program will decrease injury risk but finding a specialist to screen athletes individually is also extremely beneficial.

If I had been told about my increased risks after tearing my ACL for the first time, I would have surely tried to help decrease my chances of ending up in the condition my knees are in now, but this is the main reason I want to spread awareness, educate athletes, parents and coaches, and create quality programs for young women to use!

3.2 MEN AND THE ACL

Although men are not as high-risk for tearing the ACL as women, this doesn't mean that they are immune. Studies show that on average more men per year tear their ACL than women mostly due to the higher number of men playing sports compared to women. Women are actually most at risk for ACL tears in their teenage years due to physiological changes of the body during puberty but men are more at risk for an ACL tear from age 21-30. This age group might be more affected because of the nature of playing pick-up sports without quality strength training and conditioning programs versus younger teenage male athletes who usually play on elite teams with comprehensive training programs.

Men can also be prone to knee valgus as mentioned and described in Section 3.1.1, knee valgus occurs when the knees cave in during a load like a squat and is caused by having tight ankles, weak hips, and impaired function in the quads and hamstrings and creates extra strain on the knee. A sedentary or chair bound lifestyle is a major contributor to these symptoms, again leading to the main reason men are more at risk for an ACL tear from age 21-30 when they typically become more sedentary. Other factors like over pronation at the foot can occur in male athletes as well although it is not as prominent.

The tibial plateau is also an emerging factor relating to men and women alike regarding ACL injury incidence. As discussed in section 3.1.1 the tibial plateau is the part of the lower leg that makes up the bottom of the knee joint. It is a major weight bearing component of the body and each human has different angles in the shape of their bone that can change the way this part of the knee works. In almost all women and some men there is an increased slope angle in the tibial plateau. This increased slope causes an increase in stress to the front portion of the knee and allows it to much more easily create too much extra movement in that spot which can rupture the ACL.

It is also very interesting that in most tibial plateau studies a large percentage of women have an increased slope at the tibial plateau and only a small number of men, but of the men who do have an increased slope many of them subsequently tore their ACL. It can be said that more convincing data has been reveled from the men studied with increased tibial plateau because most all women have that deviation which is one major reason for the 2-8 time increase in ACL injury rates in women versus men.[3] The men with the deviation also have a higher risk for ACL injury than men without the deviation. X-Ray can detect the tibial plateau slope angle and further studies will be conducted on risk factors for men and women with increased slope at the tibial plateau.

Simply put, the male body was designed for activity, fighting, and protecting. Men are naturally more equipped to play sports. Because of their increased muscle mass, smaller Q angles, decreased amount of estrogen, larger and more mobile knee structure, equal ratio of quad to hamstring and glute function, and many other reasons they naturally are better equipped to avoid injury. But men, don't think you are immune. Sedentary and overweight societies in the future will further increase the ACL injury risk for men. Our chair bound lifestyles cause weak hips and weak core musculature which significantly increases injury rate and pain incidence. More simply put, when you gain weight and lose muscle function injury risk always increases.

This is even more supporting evidence for quality strength and conditioning programs and plyometric training problems do prevent ACL injuries. All athletes should keep this in mind, especially if you have already injured your ACL. Remember after suffering one ACL injury your risk of re-injury increases from 1 in 3000 to 1 in 50! Leg dominance or one leg being stronger than the other leg is very common after ACL injury which results in an increased injury risk for both legs.

4

THE ACL TEAR AND WHAT TO EXPECT

SO WHAT REALLY HAPPENS WHEN YOU TEAR YOUR ACL?

As mentioned previously most ACL tears happen during a cutting, jumping, deceleration, or in a contact movement. Typically your foot is planted firmly on the ground and a subsequent force hits your knee. This can be from contact with another player or from change of direction, quickly slowing down, or landing from a jump. Injuries can range in severity from a mild sprain to a complete tear of the ligament. Sometimes during a more intense injury an athlete can tear multiple ligaments in addition to the ACL like the meniscus or MCL. This only further decreases stability at the knee and makes for a tougher recovery.

After experiencing an ACL tear there can be a wide variety of symptoms. An ACL tear feels almost like a small rip or pinch deep inside of your knee followed by a large rush of incredible and immense pain. Some athletes fall to the floor in pain and other athletes are in such shock they attempt to keep playing and are surprised when they fall to their knees. It's fascinating how such a specific injury can have different reactions and pain severity levels for different athletes. And how even though it is a very common and easy to distinguish injury; there are many athletes with misdiagnosed ACL tears.

Many athletes hear a popping noise at the impact of injury. Some athletes are able to walk after tearing their ACL (dependent on swelling) and some aren't able to put any pressure on their leg without it buckling underneath them. Buckling or the knee giving out is a major indicator of a torn ACL. When the ACL is nonfunctional there is decreased stability at the knee joint causing it to give out periodically. Remember the analogy of the ACL as a rubber band holding your upper and lower leg together; well when the ACL tears there is no rubber band preventing your upper leg from moving too far in front of your lower leg; this is the phenomena of your leg giving out on you. There is no ACL to control the movement so the leg buckles underneath you. This is usually more prominent with going down stairs or changing directions as these are the movements the intact ACL contributes to.

Swelling is always an indication of trauma and is extremely common following an ACL injury. But usually after a few days of initial injury the swelling will go down and in most cases the athlete will be able to at least walk. It would be best to buy a basic hinge knee brace from the store so that your knee has a support system until you can make an appointment with an orthopedic surgeon. In some cases, especially when more ligaments than just the ACL are torn the athlete will be left immobilized and not able to walk. In this case, physical therapy before ACL reconstruction is going to be a key factor so that the athlete has proper strength, range of motion, and decreased swelling leading into the surgery.

If you think you might have suffered an ACL tear make an appointment with an orthopedic surgeon as soon as possible. Even if you are unsure about having surgery it is going to be essential in your healing process to see the doctor, get an MRI, and seek guidance and counsel from your surgeon on the plan that is best for you and your knee.

The initial injury is painful enough but finding out the diagnosis is a torn ACL is where the most significant amount of pain comes from. A plethora of thoughts and emotions flood your body. This is not a typical injury where a doctor can fit you with a cast and then you play the waiting game for it to heal. This is a detrimental season ending and sometimes career ending injury which usually requires surgery and a very long and tedious rehabilitation and recovery process. Your life and your knee will be forever different. It is now time to do the research to prepare yourself mentally and physically for the ordeal that you have in front of you. It's important to know that you are not alone. The ACL club and the ACL comeback story is unique to a number of courageous athletes who encounter its setbacks. You do not choose to be a part of this family of athletes but you will learn more about yourself through this injury and recovery than you ever have as a healthy individual. It is up to you and your mindset whether you let this news hinder you or whether you open yourself up to the vulnerability of your struggle to encompass change and growth mentally and physically.

4.2 HOW DO I TREAT MY TORN ACL?

Typically most ACL injuries will be treated initially with the R.I.C.E. Method, which stands for Rest, Ice, Compression, and Elevation. If you think you have torn your ACL, implement the R.I.C.E. Method immediately to ensure that pain and swelling can be managed until you are able to get an appointment with an orthopedic surgeon. Crutches might be necessary at first depending on the severity of your injury and ligaments torn. More than likely, within a few days of your ACL tear, you will be mobile enough to go about your daily life with the support of a hinge brace you can buy at the drugstore and the implementation of the R.I.C.E. Method. Keep in mind controlling your swelling is key in maintain mobility and decreasing pain while you wait on diagnosis. Remember, walking on your torn ACL will most likely feel fine, but be careful when changing directions or pivoting. This is where a common hinge knee brace will help you tremendously.

Before scheduling with an orthopedic surgeon, make sure you do your research! Don't just pick the first surgeon to come up in your network. Many orthopedic surgeons have diverse specializations and have different surgery techniques. This doesn't make them wrong or improper, but it can make a difference in the outcome of your procedure, and the longevity of your knee. Ask your friends and family for referrals. Research the surgeons' website, which will list the procedures they perform and their specialties. I recommend getting multiple opinions if you have the means to see a few different surgeons. This way, you will get a better feel for a doctor you trust and the doctor you feel has more experience in the type of surgery your knee requires.

Once you meet with a surgeon, you will more than likely need an MRI. Make sure you go to an imaging center your surgeon approves of because there can be some with poor images and poor quality. Many imaging clinics will also interpret your MRI for you. This is okay but wait until you speak with your surgeon for official diagnosis on your injury because some technicians can overlook different spots on your MRI. And if you have chosen your doctor wisely, he or she will be taking your entire physical and athletic self into consideration.

More than likely, if your ACL is torn, then your surgeon will recommend reconstructive surgery to fix the damaged ACL because the ACL is unable to repair itself. It is important to note the difference between ACL repair and ACL reconstruction. ACL repairs refers to a technique of passing stitches through the stump of the ACL but it only applies to 3% of ACL tears because most ACL tears a full rupture of the ACL requiring a reconstruction procedure using a graft to replicate the anatomical ACL. New treatment methods like platelet rich plasma injections and stem cell therapy are becoming popular, but no research proves that this option is better than reconstructive surgery. These could be potential possibilities if you lead a sedentary lifestyle, have only a partial sprain, or if timing for surgery is not right in your life. Again, make sure you discuss all options with your doctor so that you devise the appropriate plan for your knee, your body, and your life.

Surgery is not a necessity, you can function without an

ACL, but typically it is the preferred option for most active patients, because without a functioning ACL, you run the risk of developing arthritis, further damaging the knee, and the possibility of not being able to lead an active lifestyle due to your unstable knee. The more unstable your knee is the more long-term wear and tear it will receive. Think about an unstable table leg. Every time you sit at that table the legs shakes and wobbles. Eventually it has wobbled for so long the table isn't structurally sound and becomes unusable or even breaks. This is the risk you run without having an ACL.

There is also increased risk of re-injury when playing sports on a torn ACL, so make sure you consider all factors regarding your options and factors influencing your decision. Some patients are less symptomatic, or experience less pain and dysfunction with a nonfunctional ACL, and if that is the case then surgery might not be the best route for you. Any arthroscopic procedure is going to cause some level of potential arthritis risk, but living a long life without an ACL keeping your knee stable also runs a risk of developing arthritis because of the shear wear and tear forces that happen every step you take with that nonfunctional ACL. Now if you work a desk job and are very sedentary with no desire to be active then nonsurgical treatments might be the right option for you. Whatever the case, remember it is your decision and you can time it out exactly how you would like to.

Depending on your decision about ACL reconstruction and the severity of your tear, it could be highly beneficial to seek an Exercise Specialist or a Physical Therapist to guide you through proper basic strength and stretching exercises that are safe with your ACL injury and will help to keep you functional while you await surgery. Whether you have surgery or not, you do not want to lose strength, range of motion, or flexibility because of your ACL tear. It can make your surgery much harder to approach and recover from, and if you opt out of surgery it can make your rehabilitation journey a much longer and more challenging route.

Chapter 9 details and explains a few key rehabilitation exercises crucial to master after your ACL surgery. These same exercises are very beneficial to start preforming before surgery or even if you choose not to have surgery. ACL injury can change the functional capabilities of your legs so the sooner your swelling and pain have decreased then the sooner you can start your rehab exercises. These moves set you up to remain functional in preparation for surgery, regain function after surgery, and maintain function if you plan to postpone or skip surgery altogether.

4.2.1 ATTITUDE: THE CHOICE IS YOURS

So you tore your ACL. This is going to be with you for the rest of your life and it's going to increase your chance of re-injury for the rest of your life; it's going to try and slow you down in your athletic progressions and goals for the rest of your life; it's going to increase your prevalence of arthritis for the rest of your life. But you have two choices. Choice number one: sink into decay and let this overcome you and overpower you. Choice number two: Learn as much as you can in order to get yourself better; in order to recover, rehabilitate and come back from this surgery stronger and smarter than before. This is your chance to take what you are going through and use it to make you stronger. Which attitude choice are you going to make?

You cannot control what happens to you; life can be unpredictable. But you can control your reaction to what happens to you and your attitude moving forward. The hardest part about having a setback is replaying the moment in your mind over and over, wondering how you could have avoided the situation or what you could have done to produce a different outcome. These thoughts could cause anxiety, remember, you cannot change the past. You cannot change it, you tore your ACL, that moment is over. Today is the only thing in your control, and you have a long journey in front of you to get yourself better. Strength starts with your thoughts. Make sure your thoughts align with your dreams/goals/beliefs, because what you think turns into your actions, views, and attitude.

Don't overwhelm yourself by thinking about your entire journey to recovery either, keep your thoughts focused on today and how you can be positive and better yourself right now. Setbacks are extremely difficult but never let your setback define who you are. Pain teaches you a lesson and makes you stronger in preparation you for your future. Don't label yourself as the person with the bad knees or bad luck. Your mind can hear you! Every time you say, "I can't do that because of my knee" you are giving negative energy too much power. Your thoughts create your feelings, so if you tell yourself and others your knee is limiting you, then it will. Yes, you will have limitations during your recovery, but they are temporary.

Do not allow your mind to think of them as limitations

because it will create a new feeling of self-consciousness. This is a temporary physical limitation; do not let it create a long term self-conscious feeling. You will literally be preempting yourself to be self-conscious of your knee. You have so many forces going against you in this recovery journey; you do not need yourself and your thoughts going against you too! Instead, correct those thoughts. Try saying things like "I can't do it right now but I'm working hard to be able to do it soon." Think of yourself as the person who turned their weakness into strength, or the person who had the strength to recover from a major injury, or the person who, despite being terrified to approach this journey, had the strength and courage within themselves to get through it and recover. This event has changed your life and you cannot change that so accept it and focus your mind on continuing your journey in a new direction, in a positive way.

You can overcome this setback and it will make you stronger. Take each day for what it is, and focus on your mindset in the moment. One day you will look back and be surprised and proud of yourself for everything that you have accomplished! Mindset is everything.

5

ACL RECONSTRUCTION

Here's the issue; over 100,000 ACL reconstructions are performed in the U.S. alone every single year but these reconstructive surgeries have only really been implemented since the 1970s. With only 40-50 years of long term outcome studies and the rise in female participation in sports sprouting in the 1990s causing thousands of ACL injuries for people under 25-years-old; we really are not proficient enough in providing a long-term solution to these athletes who have torn their ACL.

ACL reconstructions have become very common and because of the contact nature in men's sports and the increased risk of ACL injury in female sports we are seeing more ACL injuries than ever before. Unfortunately, the bad news is that the long-term repercussions of this procedure are slowly surfacing as the athletes from the 70s and 80s are aging and seeing long term arthritis problems and as the athletes from the 90s are entering their 20s and 30s the amount of cases with graft failure, arthritis, and meniscus tears down the road are steadily increasing.

What's worse is many surgeons have different preferred techniques for ACL reconstruction and because they don't keep track of their long-term outcome studies appropriately or their patients with complications go see other surgeons; many surgeons don't realize that many of the long-term outcomes of their reconstructions are poor. This can include anything from a re-injury to arthritis, joint laxity, meniscus tears, and even failure of the graft.

All of these issues are very significant to my life as I've had four ACL revision surgeries off of only two initial ACL injuries. In December I will have had a total of eight surgeries and I am not even 30-years-old yet. I have not played sports or even gone running since I was 14-years-old. Many of the athletes that I have met over the years have encountered similar problems with their ACL journeys so I knew that there had to be a better way to approach these injuries and surgeries and that a major change needs to be made in the industry in order to prevent other athletes from suffering the same fate as me.

Dr. Tom Myers, Orthopedic surgeon in Atlanta, Georgia, saw these same flaws with the procedures when he was doing his sports medicine fellowship and in 2003 he came up with his own version of the ACL reconstruction because with all of his research he found major technique problems in the current surgery methods and wanted to design something with a better long term outcome for his patients.

The problem is many people who tear their ACL find a

surgeon that is in their insurance network and without doing research or interviewing the surgeon just trust that he or she will give them an A+ surgery. "They think this is a surgeon and he or she went to medical school and has training and has great knowledge of the operations and I'm sure 100% of his or her patients get back to playing sports. I'm sure that 100% of his or her patients rehab in six months and I'm sure that there is no chance for re-tear or re-injury. The idea that it's actually not 100% is sometimes surprising to people. And it's not something that orthopedic surgeons will talk about when they are first meeting somebody and signing them up for surgery" *Dr. Tom Myers.*

It is important to know that the surgeon you select for your surgery has a tremendous impact on the long-term longevity of your knee. Many athletes do not return to the same level of play as before the surgery and this all has to do with the way your surgeon performs your operation. Many people believe ACL surgeries are common and easy to comeback and return to sport because of some of the famous athletes' comebacks but this is not always the case. Even so, many of these famous athletes are able to play a few more years in their sport but 10 years down the road have many complications due to the nature of their surgery and how it was executed. This is never reported in the media. Again, we are just now learning and studying the learn term effects because this is a relatively new procedure.

"Even in high level with published data, the return to play rate (meaning you play at least one snap in the NFL) is somewhere around 63%, which means that 27% of these athletes never play another down in the NFL. They blow their ACL and they never come back. These are supremely conditioned athletes with the best physical therapists and the best trainers with the best rehab and genetically they are specimens and for 27% of them it's a career ending injury" *Dr. Tom Myers*.

5.1 WHAT TO EXPECT

5.1.1 Short Term

Surgery for ACL injuries involves reconstructing or repairing the ACL. ACL Reconstruction uses a graft, a section of tendon either from your leg or from a deceased donor, to replace the torn ACL ligament. The procedure is usually performed arthroscopically which means it is done with small incisions to allow surgical tools into the joint and to hold a tiny tube like video camera (the arthroscope.) Your surgeon will drill tunnels in your femur or upper leg and in your lower leg or tibia. These tunnels are used to help anchor the graft in the correct position which is secured to your bones by screws or other fixation devices. This replicates the ACL and allows your new graft to grow as a replacement. If the tunnels are drilled improperly then the graft will be more susceptible to failure.

Ask the Expert – Dr. Tom Myers elaborates on ACL reconstructions and the issues regarding poor placement of the graft and improper angles of the tunnels:

"If you're looking for the single most studied and proven chance of a poor outcome for this surgery it has to do with poor placement of the tunnels. The biggest mistake that we are making is that we are missing the attachment site of where the ligament used to attach."

In most cases, general anesthesia is used and you will be unconscious for the procedure. Most surgeries are out-patient so after recovering from anesthesia and any side effects, you will be sent home. At this point you will still have many of the medications from surgery in effect so you will be in pain, but expect day 2 -3 to be much more painful when those drugs wear off. *Warning!* Days 2 and 3 will most likely be the absolute hardest regarding pain so be prepared with tips provided in the upcoming sections. It is essential to go straight home and work on your three primary focuses for the next few days and weeks: ice, rest, and staying on top of your pain medications. The surgery might leave you feeling nauseous or not in the mood to eat but it is important to hydrate and eat some healthy hardy carbohydrates so that you can take your pain medicine regularly and keep them down.

Pain tolerance varies and there are also variations to receiving pain relief after surgery. There are options of having a nerve block to temporarily numb the leg or even a pain pump inserted into your leg allows you to manually pump medicine directly into the knee. The first two surgeries I had were Patella Tendon Autografts. During recovery if I tried to move my leg after elevating it, the rush of blood to my knee felt like someone had stuck a butcher knife directly inside of my kneecap and left it there. As I crutched to the bathroom it felt like someone grabbed that butcher knife and turned it around in my knee. This is why it is so important to follow icing, elevating, and pain medication protocol after surgery and to allow blood flow to gradually return to your knee before moving it. In comparison, my cadaver allograft surgeries were still extremely painful but honestly it wasn't comparable to the pain felt from the patella tendon graft procedure. In retrospect though, the patella tendon graft surgeries should have left me with more stability for the tradeoff of the increased pain levels had my surgeon not inserted my ACL graft at the wrong angle.

For the first one to three days it is important to get as much rest as possible. It is best to plan on staying in your bed or on your couch for at least 5-7 days. The surgery will leave your knee very swollen. Your biggest priority in week one is the ongoing management of your swelling! Why? Swelling is the main cause of atrophy or muscle loss after surgery. The more swollen you are, the more your muscles will weaken and stop firing, and the less range of motion you will have. The less muscle and less range of motion at your knee and leg; the harder, longer, more strenuous, and more painful it will make your recovery! Symptoms of swelling could last up to a month or longer so make sure you are always prepared even as you make your way back to school or work. Ice and elevation are very beneficial and a necessity to manage your swelling but so is decreasing your activity. Don't make the mistake of trying to do too much at once even if you are feeling a little better. Most of the time this leads to overdoing it and most always leads to an increase in swelling, which slows your progress down.

Ideal protocol calls for twenty minutes of ice followed by forty minutes without ice to allow blood flow back to your knee. Repeat this every single hour while elevating your knee above heart level as much as you can. Avoid putting ice directly on your skin; use a layer of clothes, washcloth, or even a paper towel to provide a small barrier. You cannot ice too much during your recovery. Reference the ice, rehabilitation, and bathroom chart in section 9.1 for ideal timing to prevent swelling and prevent the pain experienced when moving your knee from an elevated position. It will make a huge difference!

To prevent swelling at the feet and ankles, make sure you routinely move your toes around and move your ankles and feet in circles and side to side. It's important to keep the swelling down but you don't want you to lose feeling in your feet or ankles. The elevation and ice will not only help with swelling but also pain management. When you attempt to get up and use the restroom or reposition yourself remember the sudden rush of blood to your knee is going to be extremely painful! To prevent this immense pain, make sure after elevating your knee, bring your leg down below heart level in short and slow phases. This will promote gradual blood flow back to the area, which will still hurt, but it will be much more comfortable than the sudden rush of immense pain! *Note: See Chart listed in Section 9.1*

All of the sedentary time after surgery and time spent elevating one knee can cause you to get aches and pains in other places too, like in the hips, low back, or neck. To prevent getting other aches and pains change your positioning as often as possible. The longer you are stuck in one position the more your body will adhere to it and create problems in other areas resulting in tightness or pain. Think about what position you are in when you elevate and ice your knee. Either seated or laying down with one leg above heart level and the other leg in a comfortable position.

This can actually throw your pelvis out of alignment because of the prolonged periods of time with one leg up and one leg down. It might not seem comfortable at first, but try to elevate both knees when you are elevating the injured knee. This will keep your hips neutral, and in the same position, hopefully providing a decrease in tension in your back. It will also help to practice good posture. Practice good posture by keeping your head neutral, keeping your shoulders back, and by squeezing your glutes periodically. This can be done seated or laying down. Periodically squeezing your glutes will help to keep them engaged allowing blood flow to the area and decreasing tension from your hips and low back.

Reference Section 9.1 for more detailed information on beginning your rehabilitation safely from your home and in conjunction with your physical therapist to ensure you will have a speedy and healthy recovery. This section is merely a preface for what you will be going through.

Tip! Begin taking stool softener immediately after you return home from surgery. Remember that your body is in defense mode and will be decreasing the function of certain things in order to promote a safe healing process. It's better to be safe than sorry regarding this aspect.

5.1.2 LONG TERM

ACL reconstruction is invasive and takes time for the ligament to properly heal. Time on crutches can be anywhere from two weeks to eight weeks, depending on the specificity from the surgeon or repair to damage of other ligaments during the surgery like the meniscus or MCL. A proper rehabilitation program should start a few days after surgery and take you all the way to leading a full and active life. This can mean anywhere from six to twelve months, depending on training intensity and return to sport dedication of the athlete. These timelines can vary based on progressions of individuals. Younger and stronger people typically have more of an advantage in the recovery process and can have a much faster timeline. While many studies show the ACL is not fully healed until twelve months after reconstruction surgery, many surgeons will allow certain athletes to play sports again in as little as six to nine months, again depending on how fast they progress, and the type of procedure.

Long term effects of surgery include weakness, loss of range of motion, pain, and possibility of arthritis and decreased stability of the knee. With any surgery, there poses a risk of developing arthritis later in life, but without repairing the ACL your knee joint will be put through more wear and tear long term and will most likely have the same arthritic outcome. It's important to remember not all ACL rehabilitations successfully return the athlete to the same level of play as before the surgery. Many athletes do return to the same level of play and many do not. There are tons of factors that go into these outcomes including mindset, dedication to recovery, expertise of the rehabilitation program, and other factors like the athlete's biomechanics and outcome of initial surgery. The guidelines in this book provide you with detailed knowledge on how to have the most successful surgery and rehabilitation possible. Other long time side effects include increased risk of another ACL injury; focusing on an enhanced and devoted recovery program will be key in eliminating these risk factors.

5.1.3 ACL RECOVERY TIMELINE

1-2 weeks Post-Op – This is when you will have the most pain, swelling, and tissue trauma. There will be no weight bearing during this time, so plan on using your crutches and limiting your movements as much as possible to avoid excess swelling. You should be seeing a physical therapist within one to three days of your surgery.

2-6 weeks Post-Op – Slight weight bearing will begin as tolerated by pain and doctor permitting. You will still be wearing your surgical brace for the extra protection. Continue to limit mobility; avoiding inflammation and swelling is crucial. Depending on which leg is injured, you might be able to begin driving again during this time. Continue to work on range of motion, flexibility, and basic strength exercises.

6 weeks – 3 months Post-Op – As pain and swelling decrease and strength increases you may be permitted to remove the brace and start low impact cardio move like walking, rowing, and swimming. Around three or four months your physical therapist may release you to start jogging again. Make sure you do not begin to jog if you have an altered gait pattern, you might end up causing yourself further pain. Progressions are different for each individual.

3 months – 8 months Post-Op – This begins the integration of returning to your sport. Your physical therapy will begin to get harder and more athletic based. Some surgeons will allow you to begin playing sports again around six or eight months but it depends on the surgeon and the individual progress. Allow yourself proper time to return to your sport. Extra time spent rehabilitating will only help decrease your risk of re-injury long term.

"Re-injury risk was reduced by 51% for each month after nine months of post-op recovery for return to sports" *Br. J Sports Med* 2016.

5.2 THE FIRST 2 MONTHS ARE THE MOST IMPORTANT

One of the most influential and important things Terry Trundle taught me was that the first two months following an ACL reconstruction are the most important and best indicators of the longevity of your knee. Think about it, in the first two months of ACL recovery, you should regain full range of motion and partial strength back in order to be very close in the rehabilitation process to returning to normal function. This doesn't mean you are ready to return to sport but two months is where you begin to integrate harder exercises into the training regimen and start making major progression in recovery. Your progress in the first two months sets the tone for the rest of your recovery. If you are behind in any way it could delay your recovery process and even decrease your chances of making a full recovery. The longer your leg is immobilized, the harder it will be to change and regain function. Make sure that you are prepared mentally and physically immediately following your ACL surgery to dedicate your life and time to your recovery.

It is important to rest as much as possible during the first two months to avoid excess swelling and pain from overuse. As a high school student I learned this the hard way. I was very stubborn and refused to let a surgery and crutches keep me from living my life. I wanted to attend high school football games and even attend our exciting Physics Field Trip to Six Flags of Atlanta. We had worked very hard all year in Physics class with the end goal in mind of spending an exciting day with our friends at Six Flags. One of my ACL surgeries was scheduled about two or three weeks before the physics field trip. I decided that I wasn't going to miss out on this fun event but little did I know what lingering effects it would have on my recovery.

My mother advised me not to go but I stubbornly joined my friends on the bus and headed to Six Flags of Atlanta. It was very exciting at first; everyone wanted to be in my group because I would get handicapped access to all of the rollercoaster rides which meant no waiting in line. I had money ready to rent a wheelchair when we got into the park but I didn't realize that the buses would park so far away from the entrances of the park and that worse, the place to rent wheelchairs wasn't even at the front entrance of the park but a further distance away.

We unloaded off of the bus and I started crutching my way towards the park on the hot Atlanta concrete. It was excruciatingly difficult in the hot sun and I become tied very quickly attempting to hold my leg up with the tiny miniature piece of quad muscle that I had left. Luckily one of my guy friends volunteered to give me a piggy back ride the rest of the way which was not easy for him in the heat either. I rented a wheelchair and watched all of my friends have a blast on the rides because I was unable to get on them. It was so much fun in the moment but when I got home I was miserably exhausted and my knee was literally the size of a small basketball. It took me days to get the pain and swelling to go down and when I went to my physical therapy appointment later that week Terry scolded me.

He reinforced the fact that my increased swelling only decreased my ability to fire my muscles and that my stubbornness had only lead me to have a more difficult journey in the upcoming weeks. My advice to you is to do the best you can to stay involved in your life but do not let a temporary fun event inhibit your progress. Graduations and weddings are one thing and I understand those are things you will not want to miss but is taking a class field trip really worth it in the long run? Always think twice and proceed with caution even if you are six to eight weeks out from surgery. You are still in a vulnerable spot and your body needs the time and support in order to heal.

5.3 TYPE OF PROCEDURE AND GRAFT OPTIONS

There are a few very different types of ACL reconstructions and it is important to be educated on the different types before you visit your doctor. You will want to have a meaningful conversation about the best option for you and your body. There are many factors when making the decision on the type of graft to use for your surgery and having an objective conversation with your surgeon is the best place to start. It is important to find a surgeon that will look at your case individually and not just force a surgery on you because it is their special procedure. Factors like size of the athlete, severity of the tear or tears, laxity of ligaments of the athlete, and activity level of the athlete all play into making an educated decision on graft type. As started in Section 5.2 most all ACL surgeries are now performed arthroscopically which means the incisions are small, one incision is used for a camera and one incision is used for the instruments and surgery tools. The surgeon will offer choices for the graft choice and talk through the pros and cons of each option but the decision is yours. Education of the knee needs to become your passion so that the decision of graft choice and placement is successful long term.

There are two types of grafts used for ACL surgeries; autografts and allografts. An autograft is a tendon or muscle harvested from your own body and used to replace the torn ACL ligament. Many times surgeons will use the patella tendon or the hamstrings tendon. An allograft is a tendon harvested from a cadaver and used to replicate a new ACL. There is a slightly increased risk of failure for cadaver grafts due to the formaldehyde used to clean the cadaver and due to possibility of the body rejecting a foreign tissue. In some cases, the cadaver graft will slowly fail over time and end up disintegrating inside of the knee because it never adhered to your tissue. Because of these reasons, it would be safe to avoid allograft ACL tissues unless there are special circumstances like the chance there is no way to harvest your own tissue through an autograft because of having multiple previous surgeries.

There are no shortcuts for any one of these grafts.

5.3.1 PATELLA TENDON AUTOGRAFT

Patella tendon autograft is an ACL procedure were the patella tendon is used as a graft option for the ACL. The incision is usually a two or three-inch vertical line running right down the middle of the knee cap or patella tendon. This procedure typically has better outcomes for patients with a greater degree of knee laxity (typically females in their teens.) It uses two bone plugs, which means there are two screws used and screwed into tunnels drilled by the surgeon. These bone plugs secure the ACL into place. There is an increased risk of stiffness associated with patella tendon autograft procedures and reported cases of post-operative patella pain and pain when kneeling down. This type of graft is recommended for patients with increased laxity in the knee.

-My first two ACL surgeries were performed using a patella tendon autograft. I didn't realize it then but the surgeon literally removes a piece of your patella tendon (or kneecap) and uses that boney tendon to act as your new ACL. This simple doesn't make sense because it is not even the same consistency or flexibility of a normal ACL. It is much harder so why would surgeons prefer this technique? After thirteen years, I still have a small hole in my patella tendon on each knee where the surgeon removed this tendon.

It is very painful and very uncomfortable for me to kneel down. For a few years in high school I had a bottom locker. I attempted to kneel and crouch down to get my books in and out of my locker. It was excruciatingly painful and sometimes I would get stuck down there unable to stand back up. I eventually stopped using my locker and carried all my books around with me because it was too painful to bend down. Unfortunately, after thirteen years of this healing, I am still in the same pain when I try to kneel down.

5.3.2 HAMSTRING TENDON AUTOGRAFT

The hamstring tendon autograft is a great procedure because the hamstrings are very resilient and typically recover quickly from being harvested as a graft. Typically, a two or four strand tendon graft is used with zero bone plugs so it is a little less invasive compared to the patella tendon autograft. Because of this there are usually fewer reports of pain and less post-operative stiffness. This procedure has a smaller incision and is usually associated with a faster recovery. Contra-indications include MCL tear or MCL laxity at the time of surgery and patients with intrinsic ligamentous laxity and knee hyperextension of more than 10-degrees may have increased risk of post-operative hamstring graft laxity. Basically meaning, athletes with more laxity at the knee might continue to have increased laxity symptoms after using a hamstring tendon autograft.

-The most resilient location to harvest a graft. Soreness will last a few weeks but the hamstrings have a unique ability to regain strength because they are not associated with being an extensor muscle needed heavily in all movements. With all the research I have done for the past thirteen years the hamstring tendon autograft is the surgery I wish I had gone with the first time I had surgery. I wish I had known back then what I known now and I wish I hadn't been so trusting of all of my previous surgeons. They all have opinions on which graft type is better but never truly helped me to decide what graft was better for me and my knee long term. I will be using a hamstring tendon graft in my next ACL surgery. Surgery number 7 will finally be done correctly with the best graft choice possible. I am very thankful for that.

5.3.3 QUAD TENDON AUTOGRAFT

The Quad tendon autograft is a relatively new procedure developed because of the much smaller incision typically located above that knee at the quadriceps tendon. This procedure was designed for patients with already failed ACL reconstruction surgeries and uses one bone plug. There is typically a higher associated for pain and the procedure is usually recommended for taller and heavier patients. But in some cases, this procedure could be beneficial to a quad dominant female athlete because it would decrease the risk of having problems associated with hamstring firing patterns during recovery. On the flip side, many female athletes are quad dominant but after having multiple ACL surgeries have a long history of VMO impairment (decrease in strength of small muscle in the quads caused by knee surgeries) which might be a contraindication to having an option that could further effect firing patterns and strength at the quads. This is why it is so crucial to gain knowledge on these grafts before discussing your options with your doctor.

-Quad Tendon Autograft is becoming very popular but I don't understand why. Because the graft in this procedure is harvest from your quads, your quad muscles will shut down for at least 6 months making rehabilitation return to sport very difficult. The quads are extensor muscles and are the primary muscle group used in many movements we perform in sport and in normal life. Because the neurological response to the quad muscles shuts down for so long after this surgery, the risk of injury when returning to sports too soon is much higher and it will be much hard to lead a normal life soon after surgery because your walking gait patterns and other movement patterns will be altered due to those extensor muscles being so weak.

One of my friends on social media had a quad tendon graft and was getting ready for her high school prom. She felt so self-conscious because her quad muscle was so flat that you could see the difference even while wearing her dress. She was extremely discouraged with her choice in graft type because she thought as a quad dominant female it would be easy to regain strength. She had fallen down the stairs many times due to her lack of strength and ending up skipping her high school prom altogether because of her associated weakness.

5.3.4 ALLOGRAFTS (CADAVER)

Allografts are associated with a 46% failure rate 4-6 years post-operative according to Dr. Tom Myers. This type of procedure became very common for most surgeons because it is much less invasive then harvesting a tendon from the patient which decreases pain associated with surgery and speeds up recovery time. It also allowed for a much quicker procedure meaning less likelihood of complications and giving the surgeon time to fit in more operations in one operating day. With increased post-operative research on higher failure rates, many surgeons are opting to refuse the allograft surgery for most patients unless there is no way to harvest an autograft for the patient.

This can happen in many cases, such as patients who have already had multiple failed autograft procedures leaving the surgeon less options of an autograft to safely harvest or possibly in a much older patient who will not need to ACL to function as long and might have health complications requiring a quicker surgery and recovery. When dealing with older patients requiring ACL reconstruction, allograft is usually a better option because of the less invasive nature of the procedure.

Allograft failure rates are much higher in people under age 25. In talking about the comparison of autograft and allograft surgeries in patients under 25-years-old, "Re-operation and revision ACL reconstruction rates (30.8% and 20.5%, respectively) were much higher for patients 25 years of age or younger than for patients older than 25 years. In our cohort of NCAA (National Collegiate Athletic Association) Division I athletes, the revision ACL reconstruction rate was 62% for allograft ACL reconstruction and 0% for autograft reconstruction."[6]

5.3.5 NATIVE DOUBLE BUNDLE

The basic idea behind the anatomic double bundle reconstruction is to reproduce the native anatomy of the ACL which you learned in Chapter 2.2 has two anatomical bundles. Each bundle has a different amount of tension when bending or straightening the knee and when just using a single bundle ACL reconstruction the reciprocal tension of these two bundles is lost. This procedure is associated with restoring better knee kinematics when compared to the other single bundle procedures. The graft used can vary based on the surgeon. This procedure is done by identifying the femoral and tibial insertion sites of both the anteromedial and posterolateral bundles and the implemented bundles can match the measured dimensions of the patients native ACL.

-Dr. Tom Myers of Myers Sports Medicine and Orthopeadic Center in Atlanta, GA is one of only two surgeons in the entire world to perform the native double bundle ACL reconstruction. He is revolutionizing the industry and I cannot wait to finally have the best choice of graft and the best surgery technique for my knee even if it took seven tries. Dr. Myers is different than any surgeon I have worked with, and that is a lot of surgeons! He doesn't have a nurse or a physician assistant to see his patients, he knows how important the doctor patient relationship is because every case he sees is different. The quality of care for surgeons is dramatically going downhill but Dr. Myers is changing the game for the world of knees.

5.4 WHAT DO I ASK MY SURGEON?

Because each patient and every injury is different knowing the types of grafts and discussing the pros and cons of each procedure, as well as the long-term side effects is extremely crucial. Write down a list to bring with you to discuss all options with your surgeon and have questions ready regarding each type of surgery and it's benefit to you as an individual. If your doctor doesn't take the time to discuss all options with you then you need to find a new doctor.

Which graft option is best for my injury and my body? Do you have outcome studies regarding my procedure and your previous patients? Which graft will give my knee the most stability? If we repair the ACL, will the MCL and meniscus heal on their own? Which graft has a better outcome for return to my favorite sport? Why is this graft option better for me than another?

And if it is your second or third ACL surgery make sure you ask questions associated with your risk of re-injury or graft failure. How many tunnels will be drilled in my knee after my second surgery? How will this affect the possibility of another ACL tear requiring another surgery? The last graft on my knee failed, how will this graft create a better long term result? Because I have a history of ACL graft failure, what is the most secure graft for my degree of ligament laxity? Why?

Do not be afraid to question your surgeon. They need to

consider you as an individual and make you feel safe and secure regarding your surgery options. Make sure the graft is appropriate for your body and your injuries. Ensure your surgeon is thinking of the best option for you, and not the best option for them fitting in as many surgeries into one day as possible. You have the right to have a full understanding of what you are going to experience and if you do not feel comfortable with your surgeon or the answers he or she gave you, then seek multiple opinions. Do your research. This is not something to take lightly.

Make sure you ask your surgeon the following:

- How many of these cases they do per year?
- Are they sports medicine trained?
- Did they do a fellowship where they learned how to do this operation?
- Do they have any long-term outcome studies on their ACL reconstruction?
- How do they drill the tunnel? Anatomically or just the way they prefer to drill?

ASK THE EXPERT: DR. TOM MYERS WITH MYERS SPORTS MEDICINE AND ORTHOPEDICS IN ATLANTA, GA

How do you know if you have selected a skilled surgeon specializing in ACL reconstruction?

"One of the problems that we have is that the average surgeon that does these reconstructions does about 10 a year. It has a lot to do with the demographics of how the orthopedic surgeons are spread out throughout the nation. It has to do with the fact that there are a lot more rural doctors that are just general orthopedic surgeons and that the ACL is treated as a common orthopedic injury that most doctors can handle. It's been show in the total joint literature and other realms of orthopedics that we need to do somewhere between 30 and 50 cases a year to become a specialist or an expert or have your skillset even be reasonable. So, doing 10 a year you're not really improving your skillset and if that's the average number of cases that the orthopedic surgeons are doing then were probably not getting A+ ACLs."

What questions should patients ask to ensure they will have a quality procedure?

"If you're looking for a surgeon to do this you might want to ask how many of these cases they do per year. You might want to ask if they are sports medicine trained and if they had a fellowship where they learned how to do this operation because they're much better at doing a good job then those who are generalists and don't have the extra fellowship training. A specialist in sports medicine will do somewhere between 30 to 50 ACL reconstructions per year."

What is the significance of the placement of the tunnels and the anatomical replication of the ACL graft?

"If you're looking for the single most studied and proven chance of a poor outcome for this surgery it has to do with poor placement of the tunnels. The biggest mistake that we are making is that we are missing the attachment site of where the ligament used to attach. The data shows that if you have a poorly placed or not anatomic graft your chance of having a meniscus tear in 10 years is upwards of 60%. The chances of having radiographic signs of arthritis in ten years are 85%. If someone does an ACL surgery on you when you are 18-years-old and sends you away for ten years; there is a 6/10 chance that you are going to come back before then with a meniscus tear. There's an 8/10 chance that X-ray will show arthritis at 28-years-old. Fast forward another 10 years and you are bone on bone and you are looking at a knee replacement at age 38. It's not without consequence to poorly place this graft and not do a good job of reconstructing the normal knee kinematics. It has consequences down the road."

5.5 PREPARATION FOR SURGERY

ACL Reconstruction is an invasive and difficult surgery to recover from. It can be frightening, overwhelming, painful, and make you feel like you are all alone. Preparing your mind, body, and space for surgery will help change the outcome of your recovery from a negative to a positive. Approaching this type of surgery without being mentally and physically prepared is advised with extreme caution. This type of surgery has weakened even the toughest of athletes, many of which deal with depression, anxiety, and weight gain. I cannot urge you enough to seek out help amongst friends and family and even online with other people who have gone through ACL surgery. It is best to know what you are going to face head on so that you can prepare yourself to be ready for the hardships. By knowing how difficult it can be, you will hopefully be pleasantly surprised with your recovery journey through preparation with the advice and guidance from others.

Feeling alone in the recovery process was a struggle for me because your whole life feels like it comes to a halt. You cannot play sports or workout and it's very hard to resume your normal life at school or work because of your physical limitations. I didn't know anyone who had an injury like mine and back then I didn't have the benefits of finding the ACL family online for support. The biggest support system for me came from my friends. I am so lucky that they cared for me so much. In high school they signed up in shifts to spend time with me every single day while I was at home recovering. They made sure that there wasn't a single moment when I was alone. One of my friends even came to live with me for my recovery week. She slept in my bed and supported me every step of the way; watching movies with me and just being there for general support. It made me feel like I had less of a handicap because she didn't move out of the bed either. I cannot speak to how much that helped me. Other friends would drop by my house after school to bring me homework and fill me in on the gossip that I had missed at school that day. They would bring me flowers, smoothies, and even lay around with me all evening until their curfews making friendship bracelets and playing card games. At that age I was sad to miss school because I loved seeing my friends and I didn't want to miss out on anything so having their support every single day was tremendous. Remember to seek out your friends and family because your support system is so crucial to help motivate you and help you to know that you aren't alone in this journey.

The long-term effects and outcome of your surgery have a large reliance on your success with surgery mentally and physically from the moment of surgery to the first two months. If you do not focus 100% on your recovery; safely and effectively gaining strength and range of motion and decreasing pain, your setbacks in the first two months could hinder you for many months and even for the rest of your life. It might seem minor, but decreased strength, range of motion, and stiffness during the first two months of recovery only make the recovery journey even harder and more painful. If you do not regain your mobility and recruit the proper muscles to reactivate after surgery in order to gain strength, then you will most likely be faced with improper movements and mechanics for a long time if not forever.

There will be many setbacks and struggles, but being prepared will help you make the best of the situation and remain focused on having a positive, stress free, and motivated attitude. There are many factors to consider regarding your recovery timeline and they can be different for different people. It is best to prepare yourself for anything so you will be ready for any type of complication that might arise. Prepping your mind (covered in Chapter 6), is an integral part of your recovery, and your rehabilitation goals and happiness during recovery fully depend on your mindset and attitude. But you also need to make sure your body and home are ready for your procedure.

Here are some things to consider:

- Do you live alone?
- Do you have stairs in your home or apartment?
- How much time will you need off work?
- Do you have someone to cook for you or bring you meals?
- Do you need help looking after a pet or your child?
- Is your home crutch friendly?
- Is your body prepared for crutches?
- Do you have a proper ice pack or ice machine?
- Is your shower or bath tub handicap accessible?

Preparing appropriately for the surgery is essential in having a safe and easy recovery. Once you have scheduled your surgery, it is time to start planning.

5.5.1 PREP YOUR BODY

Your body is about to go through major turmoil. The anesthesia, loss of function, and loss of mobility will make you feel weak, fatigued, and a loss of endurance for up to a few weeks after your procedure. Most of the symptoms depend on how well nourished you are going into the procedure. Many repercussions are normal following surgery as your body essentially becomes very confused and tries its best to return you to homeostasis as fast as possible. Because of this some major functions might be set aside to allow your body to focus on other more important areas. Constipation, irregular menstrual periods, nausea, insomnia, weight gain, fatigue, depression and many other side effects can occur as a result of the procedure. After surgery, your body is going to be focused solely on healing you from the trauma you endured during your procedure. The more help you can give your body the better! Eating healthy, working out, practicing mindfulness, getting enough sleep, drinking plenty of water, and staying strong and flexible are highly encouraged always but especially when approaching and recovery from a major surgery.

The first thing you should be focused on is getting yourself in shape for the surgery. Yes, it might sound ridiculous because you are about to be extremely sedentary while in recovery mode but the more fit you are going into your surgery the easier your recovery will be. If you are at a healthy weight and body fat percentage great, make sure you keep it that way! But if you are even slightly overweight it will make everything you do much more difficult. Getting yourself down to a healthy weight and body fat percentage will aide in your health going into anesthesia, it will make your life on crutches more manageable, and provide some relief to your uninjured leg will that have to be doing the majority of the weight bearing following the operation.

Aligning perfectly with your goal of maintaining a healthy weight pre and post op, eating a variety of healthy foods like vegetables, fruits, lean meats, eggs, healthy fats, and lots of water is extremely essential leading up to your procedure (more information can be found in Chapter 7 on Nutrition.) Eating healthy foods in lots of varieties instead of eating foods found in packages or bags is, of course, a goal even when you aren't facing ACL surgery, but now it is much more crucial. Remember you are what you eat.

Your body is made up of millions of cells are working at all times to provide you with energy, oxygen, blood supply, and more. Those cells are made of the foods you eat so think about it like this: would you want to face a major surgery filled with slow moving non-nutrient rich cells made up of pizza and donuts? Or would you be safer, feel better, and recover quicker from eating healthy nutrient dense foods before and after surgery?

Gaining strength before surgery is vital. The initial injury has probably left you weak and stiff. It might seem like the last thing you want to do is implement a strength training routine, but it is highly suggested to be as strong as possible going into the surgery. The stronger you are leading up to your surgery, the easier it will be for you to regain strength in your muscles following the procedure. Swelling is one of the main causes of weakness to your leg muscles so you will most definitely see a significant loss of strength in your surgical leg, especially in your quadriceps after the injury and after the surgery. Muscles have muscle memory and will recover more quickly after being predisposed to strength training. Chapter 9 teaches you how to preform safe rehabilitation and strengthening methods for your ACL recovery. Reference this section as soon as the pain and swelling in your knee from the initial injury are gone. Begin with the first section and advance yourself slowly according to your individual strength. Make sure that none of the exercises cause you pain. If they are painful, you might have either advanced yourself too quickly or it might be an exercise you should skip altogether.

Additionally, upper body strength will be a very important part of your preparation work so that you will be ready for your crutches. Even after injuring your ACL, it is safe to perform upper body workouts to maintain strength and prepare your body for using crutches. Start incorporating an upper body strength training regimen at least two times per week leading up to your surgery. Bodyweight training can be very beneficial to prepare yourself for holding up your body weight on crutches. Try moves like push-ups, pull-ups, seated rows, triceps dips, and planks. You could hire a personal trainer to help you with this or do research online regarding safe strength training moves if you are unfamiliar with weightlifting. YouTube and Bodybuilding.com can help or visiting blog sites of accredited trainers. Make sure any strength training you are doing is safe for you knee and has safe progressions for your upper body.

Balance exercises are important to practice on your uninjured leg as a lot of your first month after surgery will be single leg weight bearing with crutches. If you have poor balance on your uninjured leg, you run the risk of falling while you are trying to use your crutches. It is not just crutching around when you need to be prepared but also getting in and out of the bath tub or shower on one leg, using the restroom on one leg, getting up and down from the bed or couch on one leg, getting in and out of the car on one leg. The balance exercises listed in Chapter 9 are a great place to start, on the injured knee and the un-injured knee. Your uninjured leg is going to be doing a lot of work so preparing it with balance and strength training work will better prepare you to be more functional and mobile after your procedure. Being strong in the un-injured leg, in the core, and upper body will help your outcome and make your recovery much less frustrating.

Cardiovascular strength and endurance is another often overlooked but important emphasis when facing surgery. If you are in poor cardiovascular health then your risks going into anesthesia will be much greater. By preparing your heart and lungs for difficult situations they will be stronger and more equipped to guide you through your surgery. Not to mention the fact that it will be hard for you to get cardiovascular exercise for a while following the procedure so challenge yourself to get as much in while you still can. Cardio training can help to significantly reduce stress and anxiety which is much needed during this time. Strong cardiovascular endurance will help with your future endeavors on crutches as you try to leave your home following surgery. Again, the more prepared you are before the surgery the less frustration and hindrance you will face during your recovery. Please reference chapter 9 for the best way to improve your cardiovascular endurance safely leading up to your surgery.

5.5.2 CRUTCHES: HOW TO BE A CRUTCH MASTER

Mastering crutches makes a major difference in your frustration regarding ACL recovery. Depending on the invasiveness of the surgery, you will be on crutches anywhere from two to eight weeks. You aren't going to be able to do much of anything after your surgery, but if you have a hard time on crutches, too, then you are going to be in a whole lot of trouble, mentally and physically. There is an art to crutching. After using crutches for all seven of my surgeries, I am the crutch master. I used to race kids in my high school down the hall ways; no one could believe how fast I was. I could crutch forwards, backwards, and side to side. This helped tremendously, navigating the halls of high school and the narrow pathways between desks in the classroom and isles on the school bus. I crutched with ease except for when I slipped on a water spill and fell on my butt in front of the whole high school as a freshman. The entire hallway full of people froze and just stared at me, sitting there on the ground. I'm not sure if they wanted to laugh or wanted to check on me, but no one moved and no one said a word. I couldn't get back up because my knee was too immobile and finally a big senior football player walked over and picked me up, handed me each of my crutches and walked away in silence. I was too nervous to thank him at the time, but his gesture was one I will always remember.

Becoming a crutch master requires starting with the basics: form, technique, and strength. If you have access to crutches, I highly recommend practicing on them before your surgery. Make sure the crutches are set to the appropriate height by changing the bottom portion to the pre-labeled height notches. Then measure them against your body to make sure that it is accurate. When planting the crutches on the ground underneath you, the top of the crutch should come about 2 inches below your armpit and the handle of the crutch where the hand placement goes should be level to the length of your arm. Now test out your height selections by putting your hand on the handle portion and lifting up your body weight using the crutches. The legs of the crutches should be right by your sides and not out too wide, and then underarm portion of your crutch should still be about 2 inches below your armpit with a comfortable length for your hands to hold yourself up in this position. Crutches aren't meant to go directly under the armpit, which would be extremely painful and not functional.

Now that you have the appropriate height it's time to practice crutching. The uninjured leg should be planted firmly on the ground, and you should be holding yourself up about 2 inches above the actual armrest on the crutch. Bring both crutches in front of you about a foot, while keeping your core tight, and let your body slowly swing until your foot is back underneath the crutches. By conditioning your body to hold up your own weight, you will be more mobile on your crutches. Bodyweight is heavy, so it is going to be hard to crutch distances. Practice makes this process much smoother and will make your recovery life much easier.

Ask the Expert: After seven surgeries and being on crutches for high school homecomings, proms, graduations, weddings, and family beach trips; becoming a crutch master helps you maintain a normal lifestyle. Gaining upper body strength is critical to help yourself out in this area. It is best to rest as much as possible during recovery, especially while you are on crutches, but sometimes there are life events you cannot miss. If you know you are going to be on crutches for a long day, then plan ahead and buy some anti chaffing cream to rub on the sides of your body underneath your armpits. The crutches shouldn't be touching your armpits when you crutch but with long

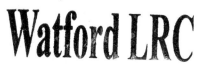

distances they can start to rub on your sides. Buy some anti-chaffing cream from a local bike shop or running shop and have it ready for those long days you can't prevent. It makes all the difference!

5.5.3 PREP YOUR HOME

This is a surgery where you will be laid up for at least a week and even after returning to work or school, will still require a lot of time resting, icing, and elevating your knee. It is important to set up your home to fit your new lifestyle to make things easier on you while you are injured. Make sure you find a dedicated recovery spot, or two. The primary spot should be where you will want to be set up for the first week after your surgery. Ideally find an easily accessible bed where you have space to have visitors, television, close proximity to the restroom, a spot to sit up and eat your food, and an area on the first floor in hopes of avoiding any stairs. A secondary spot, perhaps on a couch could also be a great change of scenery and positioning for you. At this point in the recovery, it is likely you won't have any desire to move around a lot and you shouldn't. You are in recovery mode but remember that if you sit or lay in the same position all day long you are going to get sore in other places like your back, hips, or neck. Changing positions often and even moving from the bed to the couch can help by allowing your body to shift to other positions. For more details and helping with this problem, refer to Section 5.1.1.

If you already have a pair of crutches, get them out and use them to see how difficult your home will be to navigate. Make sure you can crutch to the restroom, kitchen, or window by yourself from your recovery spot. Clean and declutter all the places in your home or apartment that you will need to access during recovery. Make common household items such as toilet paper, soap, television remote, and even water bottles easily accessible because you won't be able to carry anything while crutching. Make sure your recovery spot is not only easily accessible but has an easy way to rest and get total privacy and darkness. Think about it this way; your schedule is going to be different and you are going to be stuck in bed. You will want to find a spot that is easy to include yourself with your family, friends, or roommates, but you also want to find a location you can easily use as a quiet nap or meditation spot. Access to a window would be really beneficial. It would allow you to open the window for fresh air and hopefully get a little bit of Vitamin D. The fresh air and Vitamin D will aide your recovery efforts and also help you to feel closer to normal. Humans weren't meant to sit inside of a room all day.

Cleaning and organizing your home is crucial to creating a healthy and happy healing environment to come home to. It will help your caretaker in assisting you throughout recovery and it will help you to crutch around without obstacles in the way. It will also make your life easier over the long term because you will be immobile for a few weeks so you aren't really going to be able to clean or even clean up after yourself. It might be smart to hire a maid service for the month you are recovering or if you will rely on your spouse and family to clean, make sure they are prepared and understand their duties and most importantly you appreciate them helping you.

Don't forget about preparing your bathroom. Get on your crutches and try to use the restroom without bearing any weight on your ACL knee. Now try to lower yourself into the bathtub or get into the shower with the crutches and no pressure on your ACL knee. It is very difficult. Practicing these moves before your surgery is highly encouraged! You might feel silly practicing, but remember after your procedure you are going to be tired, weak, frustrated, and in a ton of pain, so if you have mastered your technique before the surgery then you will have a much easier time in the restroom following recovery. Be a crutch master!

Tip! At first your surgical leg will not be strong enough to lift up on your own. During my first few surgeries I had my mom lift my leg for me and help me to the bathroom. This wasn't convenient at all times and usually caused us to get in a fight because the motion would hurt me terribly and my first reaction would be to yell at her. This is not a good situation for you or for your caretaker. The best thing to do is to practice using your non-surgical leg to lift the injured leg. Bend your non-surgical leg and angle your foot underneath the ankle/calf muscle of your surgical leg. Use your arms to guide your body on your butt to easily shift and turn yourself in order to move over or to get out of bed or off the couch. This is a crucial skill to master as it will help you to remain somewhat self-sufficient.

Clean and declutter the bathroom in order to allow safe use on crutches. Remove any bathmats to avoid slipping on your crutches. It might be a good idea to find a nonslip shower mat for the inside of your shower or bath tub because you are only going to have one leg for support. You do not want to be slipping on that one leg! If you don't have a seat in your shower, then purchase a shower seat or bath pillow to provide you with support while you are bathing. Remember, you cannot get you sutures wet until after the doctor removes them so plan on having extra saran wrap in the bathroom to wrap your knee and keep it dry. Duct tape the saran wrap to your leg so no water will be able to get inside. Do not submerge your leg, but rinse off quickly so your wound will remain clean and dry.

If you don't have one already, a removable shower nozzle can be of huge help when trying to avoid getting your knee wet. It will allow you to sit down in the tub or on the shower chair and still be able to wash your hair and body while avoiding water to the knee. Another great idea would be finding a small chair to use in your bathroom, as you will have used a lot of energy showering and will need help with changing clothes.

Now that you have created your recovery zone, it is essential to get organized in the days and weeks leading up to your surgery. Making a Pre-Surgery To-Do List is what always helped me. This list should include everything you need to get done before your surgery. The list should also include any items you want to have at home to keep you comfortable and aide in your recovery. I have provided a sample Pre-Surgery To-Do List at the end of the chapter.

An ice machine and a few really good ice packs are extremely crucial both now and forever. Look for an ice machine such as the Game Ready or Active Ice, which can be purchased with a fitted sleeve for your knee. These are amazing because they give compression and extremely cold ice flowing constantly on your knee. Because you will need to change out ice packs and replenish ice in your ice machine, it is crucial to have several ice packs. The best ice packs are the larger flexible ones you can mold around your knee.

Another key item is a foam elevation wedge. After several surgeries and trying to use old pillows to elevate my knee, it is definitely worth the investment to get a foam wedge for extra support. This will ensure the wedge stays secure and that it will have enough support so there is no worry of your knee falling off. If possible get a wide enough foam wedge to support both of your legs. You won't need to be elevating the non-surgical leg but anytime you are elevating your surgery leg, remember your pelvis is slightly out of alignment in this position. It can help to avoid low back and hip pain by elevating both legs at the same time, decreasing the uneven alignment at the pelvis.

Other recommended items include a tray for your lap to help when you eat or need to do work, and a back support to help prop you up though out the day. From previous experiences, pillows are not as comfortable for back support and end up falling over. A back support with a cup holder is even better. Another great item to add to your list or possibly even borrow from a friend is a hand held back massager. You can expect to have back and neck pain from being sedentary during recovery and this device will help you stay comfortable.

Grocery shopping is best done the day before your surgery so your fresh produce and foods will last longer. Make sure you stock up on all of the essentials for toiletries, cleaning items, and any foods you will want access to during recovery. Remember, you will be on crutches for a few weeks making it really difficult to go shopping or to cook, so make sure you have friends or family available to help when preparing meals. You might try grocery or restaurant delivery services in most areas which will deliver your groceries to your door. Although it isn't the healthiest option (refer to chapter 7 on nutrition) to eat prepared or frozen meals, it might be a great option while you are immobile.

When preparing your grocery list, keep in mind that you won't be able to cook so whoever you caretaker is might appreciate an easier cooking load if they aren't very experienced. Also consider preparing a few meals the day before your surgery. You could make a healthy breakfast casserole, grill some lean fish and chicken, and even marinate and cook a lot of vegetables to have on hand. Preparing and freezing meals might also be a great option for you. No matter what, make sure you discuss your menu and cooking options with your caretaker so you can be prepared for what you both will need.

Having healthy prepared meals is a really great option but don't forget the snacks. Shortly after surgery, you might have a sensitive stomach and no appetite, quick snacks are a great way to keep your energy level up and help you to keep food in your stomach to better tolerate your pain medications. For the first few days after your procedure, it might be best to focus on foods easy to digest to avoid nausea, heart burn, and constipation symptoms. Stay away from spicy foods and acidic foods. Simple foods like bananas, oatmeal, cereal, potatoes, fruit and vegetable smoothies, cauliflower, and lightly seasoned chicken might be good examples to start with and as the days go on you will feel less sensitive and have more of an appetite.

Do you have a pet? Do you have a family member or friend willing to help you take care of this pet or do you need to set up a dog walking service or even a temporary boarding option? Make sure you have thought out options to assist you and your pet for the first month after your surgery. Cats and fish are relatively easy but if you have a dog you aren't going to be able to bathe or walk your dog for weeks and it might be difficult for you to feed your dog while on crutches too. Plan this out. Asking for help isn't easy but if you find people willing to help you before your surgery then it will be all lined up and taken care of for you.

Think ahead to all your responsibilities like carpool pick up, work responsibilities, or school requirements and talk to those who can help you in these situations. Find people to cover for you, bring home your assignments regularly, or even find a way to temporarily work from home. Again, the idea is to make your recovery as easy as possible and preparing for all of your responsibilities beforehand can really aide in stress reduction and ensuring you get the rest you need to recover.

It's also smart to plan some activities for your recovery

period. If you let your mind wander it may go to negative thoughts and bring you into a terrible cycle. Try to embrace this recovery period and use it as time to catch up on your favorite books, blogs, movies, shows, games, etc. Stock up on movies, books, magazines, coloring books or cross words so can fill this time relaxing and stretching your brain.

Keeping your mind busy is a great way to make the time go fast. It might also be good to plan to do something you are usually too busy to do. Whether it's a new book, or designing your very own website, or helping your sister find ideas to renovate her house, it helps to have a project in mind to focus your energy on. Always focus your energy on progress and positivity!

5.5.4 SURGERY PREP LIST

- Declutter home for crutches
- Deep clean home (because you won't be able to clean for a while) or enlist maid service to help you in the coming months
- Create Recovery Zone – close to bathroom, window, and away from stairs
- Grocery shopping
- Meal Prep – pre-prepared or precook foods in bulk so your caretaker won't have as much to do; healthy casseroles are a great option. Pre-grilling vegetables and meats. Freeze individual baggies of fruit for easy smoothie prep.
- Pre-buy common household items like toilet paper, tooth paste, kitchen items, or dog food. Any

items that you won't want to carry on crutches for the next few months.

- Plan on pet care or assistance
- Buy or borrow ice packs, ice machine, foam elevation wedge, electrical stimulation unit, back support device, lap tray for food or laptop, hand held massager, stool softener, acetaminophen, ibuprofen, saran wrap, melatonin, shower chair, bath pillow, bathroom chair, non-slip shower mat insert, removable shower nozzle, anti-chaffing cream for your armpits for crutching (can find at running shops or bike shops), muscle stick self-massager for tight leg muscles.
- Get coverage at work or work from home duties; find classmates to bring you school assignments, ask for help ahead of time!
- Take the trash out and recycling
- Find any books, movies, or projects you want to start on
- Do your laundry and make clothes that you will be wearing during recovery easily accessible.

6

MENTAL TRAINING

"Fear is a reaction. Courage is a decision." -
Winston Churchill

After having six previous knee surgeries you would think I'm not scared. But the truth is I'm terrified. It's really scary facing these surgeries, medical bills, constant pain, loss of movement and athletic lifestyle, and all of these uncertainties on my own. We aren't even sure if this next surgery will help because the kinematics of my knees have changed due to dealing with having an unstable knee for so many years. There are no outcome studies for us to research because there is no one ahead of me who has faced so many failed procedures. I have learned through all of this that I have to control my thoughts every single day. You have to learn to control your reaction in order to change your decision. I have to remind myself that being scared and worried about these things will not help me right now and will not help me in the future either. I choose courage. I choose positive thoughts every day. I am facing one of the hardest journeys I have been through but I have changed my life in the process by controlling my thoughts. Today is all I can control so I embrace each day with courage and an open heart.

As a stubborn athlete, the mental side of ACL surgery and recovery is the hardest part. The recovery process is long and tedious and in the moment, can seem never ending. I had different difficult struggles with each surgery, but for the most part they all sum up to feeling lost, helpless, and alone, or feeling anxious, frustrated, and mad. No one gets what you are going through unless they have gone through it themselves. Your friends and family will continue to live a normal life. Your athletic team will keep playing without you. Your sense of yourself as you formally were will be temporarily gone. You will be alone with your thoughts a lot. Thinking about why me? Why now? Why is this so hard? Why can't this heal faster? You will be alone with your recovery a lot. No one will understand the effort, pain, and dedication it will take you to get back to being an active person. No one will realize how hard it is to be left out of big events like weddings, parties, family trips, concerts, or your team's championship game.

This is why you have to learn to control your thoughts in order to change your decisions and reactions. You have to be willing to grow and learn. You have to be strong mentally in order to get stronger physically. You have to appreciate each day in the moment for anything else will cause you anxiety or fear. This is going to be a long and difficult process and I want to teach you what has helped me. I am facing my seventh knee surgery and I am terrified but I have changed my life by controlling my thoughts and you can change yours too.

6.1 MINDSET

Let's face it, surgery is a big deal and as an athlete the hardest part about your recovery journey is going to be your mindset. Active, fit, sports orientated life as you know it is now temporarily over and instead your focus will be small tedious tasks that seem to get you nowhere. No matter how young and healthy you are a surgery is still a major stressor on the body and can be very scary. With possible risks to procedures, pain, medical bills, and long recovery processes there are many factors associated with surgery that can cause some major anxiety. ACL injury and surgery can be a devastating season ending or career ending injury. Many athletes make the great comeback but many athletes also are unable to return to the same level of play as before the injury. It is very common for athletes to experience a variety of issues including anxiety, depression, loss of self-worth, or loss of self-identity. We are athletes. We give it our all out there on the field and in the weight room every day. We prepare mentally and physically for our sport. Sport is life. And when all of that is ripped from underneath you in an instant it can be extremely hard to cope with.

Many athletes associate their self-identity with their successes in their sport and losing that sport and the team they were a part of can make them feel lost, helpless, alone, and not themselves. It is important to help these athletes learn a new sense of self-worth outside of their athletic abilities. Take some of the same qualities that make them a great competitive athlete and find ways to use those in other aspects of life in order to gain confidence in other areas than just athletics. Finding support online is very helpful because no one can relate to your ACL injury unless they have been through it before. It is important to know you are not alone. The ACL family is an involuntary group of mentally tough athletes who challenge themselves mentally and physically in order to overcome the greatest of setbacks. Finding others in the ACL family will help you to remain hopeful and to have a sense of belonging other than with your team who will unfortunately continue playing without you.

It can also be helpful to join another safer sport while you are recovering or study the strategy of your sport, or film. Try things like golf, or even ping pong. It will give you something to focus on so you can channel your competitive nature into something new and positive. Remember that comparing yourself to others is not going to help you to recover any faster and it is not going to change the fact that you tore your ACL. Finding new activities will be a great compromise because building your self-worth and confidence away from your sport is the only way to remain happy and focused on the present moment during your long recovery journey.

It is totally normal for your mind to turn to negative thoughts when facing such a big event. This is a primal instinct from evolution that enabled us to survive. It's commonly referred to as your reptile brain or your lizard brain because the limbic system controlling fight, flight, freeze, and fear reactions is all a lizard's brain is comprised of. Centuries ago, when presented with life threatening situations our ancestors would use the reptile brain to control their reaction to a threat; either fight, flight, or freeze. It was survival of the fittest. Eat or get eaten. Fight or die. Now in present day the common person typically does not encounter many circumstances where they need to use their reptile brain in order to survive. But the reptile brain is still there. Now it has manifested itself into a more anxiety based reaction. We go into fight or flight mode over a car in traffic cutting us off, or as a result of receiving a bad business review. The reptile brain is taking over our reactions but we have the power to control this. We aren't lizards. We have other regions of the brain like the neocortex that have evolved into being responsible for complex thoughts, imagination, and consciousness. Humans have the power to control their thoughts which in turn will control our emotions. By controlling your conscious thoughts, you have the power to change your attitude and outcome or reaction to anything that happens to you.

All of the power to change your thoughts and your outlook on your situation comes from you. It will take conscious thought and effort to train your brain into seeing the positive outlook to everything but by doing this you will control your reptile brain with reason and logic and be able to push your anxiety and fears to the side. They will always be there though; battling for control of your emotions because of how bad that it wants you as a human to survive but you can adapt your thinking to overcome your reptile brain.

This is extremely important for everyone to work on every

day. Positive thinking takes daily work, just like eating healthy and working out. But positive thinking and mental training is a crucial piece of health that many people are overlooking or assuming that it is out of their control.

Flashback to the doctor's office; your doctor is telling you that you need ACL surgery. It is going to be costly, painful, scary, time consuming, and it will require a lot of hard work in order to recover. It isn't guaranteed that you will make a full recovery or be able to return to the activities you love. You can either let all of these negative thoughts consume you and allow your lizard brain to take over and push you into sadness, depression, and anxiousness; or you can rise above and look for the positives in order to use this setback to better yourself.

Facing surgery is going to require a lot more effort than just working on your normal day to day positive thinking. But starting now and finding the positives in every situation is a good way to start. Try writing down positive affirmations every day. Use phrases like I can, I am, and I will. Keep your list with you at all times and when your reptile brain tries to take over pull out your list and adjust your mindset back to positivity. I am strong and successful. I will make the Dean's list. I will make my comeback. I am strong enough to recover from ACL surgery. I will play soccer again. I am going to make a difference. I will get on the Ellen Show.

I began writing a list of positive affirmations down every single morning once I found out about my next round of surgeries. Every morning I focus my mind to think and live in the moment and it sets me up for a day of success and less anxiety. I have been writing these phrases down and numbering them. Today I wrote number 128. I can truly say that while facing one of the scariest and most stressful situations of my life, I have totally changed my life in the process by controlling my mindset. I have started up projects and tasks in the past 128 days that I never thought possible. I have achieved more in the last 128 days than possibly in the last 5 years of my life. Your thoughts are a powerful tool. Learning to control them to help you is extremely powerful.

Learning to appreciate everything daily and live in the moment is crucial to keeping a happy, healthy, positive mindset. Daily appreciation helps you to live in the moment and keep your mind in control of the present because that's the only place it can help you. When you let your mind wander into the past and overanalyze or drift into the future and create expectations then you are just setting yourself up for failure. This is important to remember every day but especially while you are going through your ACL surgery and recovery.

During recovery, it will be easy to accidentally rush your progress, your feelings, and even your mindset but you have to remember that living in the present is the best way to reach success. If you think about what you used to be able to do or what progress you wish you had already made with your knee, then you are going to be disappointed and being disappointed during recovery is going to slow you down. Focus on the present day and what you can do today to help you recover, mentally and physically. 1% better every day is 365% better in a year! Celebrate and appreciate your accomplishments each day, even if they seem small. I am so thankful that I was able to go on a walk today. I really appreciate finding a quiet and safe place to practice my gait patterns and help to regain endurance in my leg. I am thankful for my friends and family helping me to recover today. I am so happy to have walked up the stairs today without any help from my crutches. This helps you to live in the moment and focus on the present instead of the future or the past. It might help you to keep a journal of your daily appreciation. Writing these down and then saying them aloud will help to reaffirm your thoughts. This can also serve as a version of your proof list for later if you need to pull it out as inspiration. This goes for your knee recovery and your mindset each and every day. Learn from every single day. That's how you get better.

Having patience and accepting the present moment is crucial for your recovery journey. Patience is meant to prepare you. You cannot be content with where you are when you are more focused on where you are not. You rob your own joy. Being content with where you are today and happy with yourself today is all in your control. And until you can control that, life will never feel in control to you. It's the same thing as looking back to the past, this will only create anxiety because you cannot alter the past. The only thing you can do is focus on today. Focus on being happy today. Focus on what you can do today to prepare for your surgery or rehabilitate your knee. But today is the only thing you can control. Accept that and you will bring peace into your life.

So remember, it is still survival of the fittest. You might not get eaten by a lion but your happiness and success in this world fully depends on you and your ability to adapt to situations to enable growth versus decay. In every situation in your life your attitude will determine your direction so be smarter than the lizard. Work actively every day to control your lizard brain and let your logical and analytical side of your brain flourish!

Start listing your positive affirmation statements on the next page, and affirm, "I CAN, I AM, I WILL."

6.2 MEDITATION

As you have learned, happiness comes from within you. You are in control of your thoughts, feelings, reactions, views, and the things and people you surround yourself with. By taking control of your conscious thoughts you have the power to choose positivity and control your attitude in any circumstance. This is where true happiness lies: accepting today for what it is and realizing that the past and the future are not in your control. Facing a severe injury like an ACL tear is a complicated mental process. It will take you from shock, anger, sadness, regret, fear, anxiety. Why did this happen to me? Why did I have to take that last shot at practice? What am I going to do? Will I ever play soccer again? Can I make it through surgery? These are all common reactions but remember you have the power to change your reaction. You have to find it within yourself to remember that you are the only one that will get you through this hardship. Emotional thinking and overanalyzing your injury and surgery will only lead to negative emotions. It is hard to keep those thoughts away when facing such a traumatic event so you have to take control.

Along with the mindset training tips listed in Section 6.3, meditation is a wonderful way to take control over your emotions and destress your anxieties. You don't have to sit cross legged and channel in Buddha as you hum but be serious with taking control of your mind. Find an isolated, quiet space where you practice your meditation. Turn on some easy listening music; an orchestra, nature sounds, or the silence of a fan blowing. Find a comfortable position whether it be seated or lying flat on the ground. Now just do your best to think of absolutely nothing. Turn off your brain entirely. Breathe in deeply through your diaphragm and feel your stomach rise and fall.

It might be hard at first to shut your mind completely off. Instead practice counting your breathes, singing the lyrics to your favorite song, or reciting your I am, I can, I will statements of affirmation. Learn how to shut your mind off of negativity and control your thoughts in a positive way.

Sometimes even controlling simple thoughts like those is difficult. That was my biggest setback when I began meditating; I couldn't just shut my mind off. Instead I dedicated an hour every day to dimming the lights and practicing my breathing; and if that wasn't working then I began journaling. This is when you can get out a piece of paper and write down everything positive about yourself, your life, and your comeback story. It can be words, phases, or sketches; goals, dreams, or ambitions. Write down things that make you happy and fuel your confidence or even cut pictures out of magazines to help you visualize your dreams and positive things in your life. Visualize yourself doing these activities or read them inside your head or out loud over and over until you motivate and compel yourself so much that you are shouting with joy! I am stronger because of my setbacks. I will recover from surgery stronger and smarter. I will be happy. I will climb Mt. Kilimanjaro. I will learn how to surf. I can control my happiness. I inspire other athletes. I love my scars. I will not let my weakness slow me down. I am wonderful. I am incredible. I can do this! Even though this is not your typical form of meditation, it can still be a helpful way to control your thoughts and keep away your anxieties. By dedicating time each day for meditation, you will find the style of meditation that works for you. Work your way towards a more silenced and relaxed state because that is great healing time for your mind and body. With more practice it will be easier for you to tune out and control your emotions.

6.3 POSITIVE AFFIRMATIONS

6.3.1 For You

Practice Positive Self Talk: As a teenager, going through challenging surgeries made me very frustrated. You cannot do anything on your own and it can be very easy to take out your frustration on those around you. I had a big tendency to get angry because I couldn't do anything for myself and then get sad because I felt helpless and trapped. I used self-talk to pull myself out of this downward spiral. I finally picked myself up and told myself that this is a journey and I had to approach it day by day, step by step and crutch by crutch. I told myself "Patience, Persistence". I repeated it to myself over and over and over until I listened to myself and believed it. From then on any time that I was feeling upset or frustrated at my lack of progress or ongoing weakness and pain I would tell myself "Patience, Persistence", "What can I do right now that will help me tomorrow?" By simplifying my thoughts and focusing on the positives I pulled myself through and mastered my rehabilitation. I knew I wanted to be better, be stronger, smarter than I was before this surgery and I wasn't going to let the surgery win.

Try finding your own words for positive self-talk. Use words that inspire emotion out of you, words that make you feel compelled to be better. Repeat them over and over during tough times. Write them down. Visualize them. The more these words become a part of you the more inspired they will make you and the more you will start to believe in their power.

Practice Positive Mental Imagery: Even if you are unable to walk or squat it can help to use visualization techniques to keep your mind focused on progression and not setbacks or inconveniences. Imagine yourself walking again, squatting again, and playing your favorite sport again. Think about how happy this makes you feel and how much it will mean to you to do these activities again after having them taken from you. Imagine how great it will feel to complete your first challenging workout or getting through a tough new hiking trail. Think of how amazing it will be to dress up and go out with your family and friends again for the first time after surgery. Think of others you can positively influence through what you learn during your setback. Picture yourself achieving a new weight loss or strength goal. Imagine going on a trip of a lifetime with your new knee aiding you to new discoveries.

The bottom line is there will be times during recovery that you don't know if you can keep going. You will be frustrated and upset with the fact that you are stuck in bed and immobile. You will be sad about losing strength and feeling very weak. You will feel left out from the outside healthy walking world. This is why it is so important to bring your mind away from this place; away from all of the negativity, because negativity attracts more negativity. You will have to visualize a new place in order to escape the negative. Remember mindset is your biggest tool.

Set Safe and Realistic Goals: This will help to keep you in control of your anxiety. If you take control then your anxiety will take the backseat. Setting safe and realistic goals can help you to stay motivated on your tedious day to day tasks during rehabilitation. Your goal week 1 out of surgery should be controlling the swelling. Maybe you set a goal with your physical therapist regarding your single leg balance exercises. It's also important to make goals about everything though, not just rehabilitation based. Short term recovery goals and long term recovery and life goals help you to focus on the process in the moment so that your mind will not be thinking of anything negative or anything outside of its control. Think about a dream trip you want to take or a new skill that you want to learn. Having something to look forward to helps keep your mind on the positives! And a healthy mind will help you to progress your recovery in order to reach these goals which creates continued motivation for your cause.

Milestones are great to set as a goal to keep you focused but remember that each person and recovery is going to be a little different. Make sure that when you are goal setting you don't rush your rehab and set unattainable goals.

Keep Your Attitude in Check: Remember this takes daily practice. Your attitude determines your direction. Are you going to comeback from this surgery even stronger than before? Or are you going to feel sorry for yourself and use this as an excuse to become overweight and lazy? Don't get bitter, get better! There is so much to learn about yourself when you go through tough times so learn to embrace these lessons and grow from them. Learn to appreciate having a healthy and working body because not everyone is so fortunate. Learn to use the awful experience to teach yourself new healthy habits inside and outside of the gym. By appreciating this experience and what you learn from it, you will find that all of your struggles in the future will be a little easier to handle. Your ACL recovery journey will prepare you for something great one day. By appreciating your journey, you will be open to the possibilities of your dreams and positively directing your life towards them.

6.3.2 TO GIVE TO YOUR ANESTHESIA TEAM

For me, one of the scariest parts of the surgery is the moment you are rolled into the surgery room. First you see many scary looking machines, mirrors, tools, and devices. It looks like what might be on the inside of a UFO. Then you notice how many people are actually in the surgery room with you and immediately comes a rush of stressful emotions including the release of the stress hormone cortisol. This is it, it's about to happen. You are going to wake up and your life will be so different. Very soon after this the anesthesia team administers your medication and within 10 seconds you are out; your last memories being left with stress, anxiety, and fear. There is a better approach!

Simply ask your anesthesiologist to read off a few prepared phrases before they put you to sleep. This will help you to relax, decrease your release of cortisol, and will help to control your mind going into your procedure. What you think you become; so, if your last few thoughts before going under anesthesia are positive and powerful you will be too!

Try using reaffirming statements for a successful procedure

and recovery. Similar to your positive affirmations to use during recovery it is best to use statements with I can, I will, and I am; but word them in the third person for your anesthesiologist to quickly and easily read aloud to you. For instance, you will have a successful surgery. You will rehabilitate and comeback stronger than before. You are resilient and prepared for this surgery. You can do this.

I used this technique for my 7th surgery and along with the additional mindset training I had been doing; it made all the difference. I recovered from anesthesia feeling happy, empowered, and focused instead of in pain and nervousness. It truly was the best way I have ever felt waking up from a procedure. The mind is a powerful tool.

6.4 MILESTONES/PROOF

During rehabilitation milestones are important to celebrate and keep track of. Not only is it positive reinforcement to keep your mindset focused on your goals but it's also a great way to ensure that you will progress each and every week as expected. Celebrating your milestones is different than goal setting. By appreciating the progress you have made, it better reinforces your mind to focus on the positives in your journey and not the negatives. There is still a long road ahead and it might seem silly to celebrate your first trip up the stairs but remember appreciating the moment is the biggest key to happiness. Think about it, we celebrate many milestones in life in order to appreciate the moment; birthdays, anniversaries, graduations. Why should your ACL surgery be any different? Now you certainly don't have to throw a party for doing your first squat after surgery but this is a big milestone for you so embrace it and appreciate your progress.

Making a "proof" list in my first personal training job changed my outlook on life. I had a lot of obstacles going against me like my knees and my youth but the biggest obstacle going against me was my attitude and my perception of myself. I starting making a list of "proof" every day so that when I was feeling down I could refer to the list and remember my positive progress and why I was on my mission in the first place. Your "proof" is anything positive that happens in conjunction with your recovery. Start a daily or weekly "proof list" and when you have a bad or negative day pull out your list of proofs to use to reinforce your positive thoughts. Your "Proof list" can also be celebrated as your milestones list. This process of recovering from surgery is a long and grueling one so celebrating the milestones is a great way to keep yourself focused on the positives. Literally think of it as your proof that you are progressing. It can be hard to see your day to day progress when trying to achieve a big goal like graduating college or rehabilitating your recent knee surgery.

The big picture can be overwhelming and very easy to compare yourself to an unrealistic timeline. Add daily items to your proof list. Examples for graduating college might be: got an A on an exam, a professor took time to help you out, or you met a study buddy in class. Examples relating to your recovery from surgery might sound more like: regained full flexion in the knee, had a friend come and visit you during recovery, or had your first full night of sleep since surgery.

It can be anything big or small but it all ends up aiding in your recovery and when you have a day when you need help finding positive thoughts it's time to reference your proof board for actual proof on the positives on your journey. It's like you are compiling a list to motivate yourself with. A list of the small things that happen daily that contribute to your outcome. I recommend keeping your list on your bathroom mirror or in your car (somewhere that you see it every day) so that you will have constant reminder of your progress.

_____

_____

_____

_____

_____

_____

_____

_____

_____

_____

_____

_____

_____

_____

_____

_____

Tip! Dealing with the Knee Brace: How to Still Feel Feminine

One of my biggest struggles revolves around my knee brace. It's uncomfortable, annoying, and most of all hard to wear with anything except workout clothes. This works fine for me most days of the week as I work in a Personal Training Studio, but when I dress up, I find it difficult to find an outfit that works with the knee brace and is comfortable and cute at the same time.

During my first few surgeries I would try to hide the knee brace or refuse to dress up because it was too difficult or not worth trying. To me, the attention from the knee brace always feels negative and seems to label me so I preferred trying to hide the brace or not make social plans to avoid talking about my injuries. But I found through this journey of knee surgeries, I was letting the knee brace have control and by taking control myself I could still feel comfortable and feminine as an injured athlete.

Here are some tips that might help with dressing up in your knee brace.

- Take control. Determine what you want to wear based on comfort and your likes instead of what looks good in the knee brace.
- Don't be afraid to dress up. You have to wear the knee brace anyway. Own it. Wear the cute dress and don't worry about all of the odd looks you will get.
- Find a knee sleeve that helps avoid the brace rubbing when wearing shorts.

- Be comfortable. Don't feel pressured to wear anything you aren't comfortable with wearing. If you don't want to dress up then you don't have to.
- Choose exciting outfits that take away the focus from your brace. This is fun because if you wear something beautiful or different, you will realize that people notice you and not just your brace.
- Accessorize your brace. Jewels, flowers, stickers. Make it fun.
- EmBRACE it. Work it. Own it. You are YOU and not your brace.

No matter how large your brace is or how long you have to wear it, gain the confidence in yourself to not allow it to discourage you and not allow anyone else's comments about your brace or your injury to affect you. This is not easy. When I first started college my suite-mate saw the scars on my knees and exclaimed, "Your knees are uglier than my grandma's!" It hurt my feelings and for *years* I was nervous to wear shorts for the fear of what people would say about my scars.

It's not worth the time and emotion to allow someone to discourage you in that way. Just know that your knees and your brace do not define who are you and no matter what anyone says you are an amazing, beautiful, and unique person. People's viewpoints come from their own insecurities so never allow someone's perceptions of you to change your perception of yourself.

EmBRACE it!

Chapter Recap

• Mindset is everything. You are facing a major life event and the quality of your recovery is all based on the quality of your thoughts. Make sure they are positive.

• The most difficult parts of ACL surgery and recovery is not the physical pain; it's the mental pain. The frustration that you cannot do what you once could and that you have to start over totally from nothing in order to get back to where you want to be. Do not allow your thoughts to think about the past or the future. Think about the present day and the present moment to avoid anxiety. Do a little bit each day to reach your goals and appreciate your successes each and every day!

NUTRITION

PRE-OPERATIVE/GENERAL

Nutrition is extremely important in the functioning of your entire body. Energy is created from the foods that we eat and either used and harvested for metabolic functioning or stored as fat. Any excess calories are stored as fat whether they are from healthy foods or not. Someone with higher levels of fat is going to have a harder time recovering from ACL surgery because of the increased pressure on the knee joint, increased risk of complications during surgery, and decreased amount of muscle mass in the body. Anesthesia also binds to fat so the more fat you have the longer the lingering effects of anesthesia could be. For every one pound of additional fat on your body it is four times the force on your knee joint. If you are even ten pounds' overweight, it will aid your recovery substantially to get down to a healthy body fat percentage for your body.

Disregarding your ACL injury, nutrition should already be

a primary concern in your life to ensure that you are healthy and treating your body with the fuel it needs to lead a long life. Our bodies are made up of billions of cells, these cells live and die and operate solely from the food that you eat. Think about it. Our bodies require certain amounts of vitamins, nutrients, water, carbohydrates, fats, and proteins in order carry out every process required to keep you alive and functioning. Your skin cells are replenished from the food you eat, your energy is created from the food you eat, the functioning of your brain relies on the food you eat, and even the cartilage in your joints is created and destroyed from the fuel you provide your body. It's very simple, you are what you eat. Think about the car you drive every day and in order for your car to operate at full capacity you have to give it gas, oil changes, etc. so that it will have a greater longevity saving you money. It's the same thing with your body. You only get one body. You wouldn't want to fill it with diesel fuel when it requires normal gasoline. That is just asking for disaster. So why would you ever fill your body with excess sugar, fake food, dyes, and chemicals? You will not get a great return on your investment and this investment is your life!

The best investment you can make in your health is eating a variety of fresh fruits and vegetables, adequate amounts of carbohydrates, healthy fats, and proteins, drinking a lot of water, and eliminating sugar, processed foods, and over eating in general. If this is a challenge for you or you are unsure of the amounts of foods that you should eat, then it is highly recommended to seek guidance from a licensed dietitian or nutritionist. This will give you the proper guidance on serving sizes, food choices, and adequate intake of vitamins and minerals.

Now, back to your ACL injury. Your surgery is scheduled and a very essential part of your surgery is obviously your recovery. The healthier that you eat, the easier it will be for you to fade off the effects of anesthesia which can linger in your system for up to a few days. Also, heading into your surgery, it is very essential to have healthy all natural foods in your diet for a number of reasons; including overall effects of anesthesia, risk of surgery in general, complications from surgery, healing from your surgery, and decreasing the likelihood of side effects from surgery including blood clots and even constipation. If you eat poorly leading into your surgery, it's like preparing your car for a cross country trip without getting an oil change, having a spare tire on hand or filling up the gas tank all the way. You are destined to have a difficult trip with many roadblocks. Hopefully you make it to your destination safely.

7.2 POST-OPERATIVE/ HEALING

Remember that your recovery is essential in the longevity of your knee and by eating a healthy nutrient dense diet your body will have the proper fuel to recover quicker and more efficiently. After your surgery, your body is going to be in fight or flight mode quickly doing everything in its power to heal you from the trauma and tissue damage and ensure that you will survive and thrive. Your body is going to require adequate nutrients to remodel bone, clot the blood around your incision, build new skin cells to repair the incision, heal the scar long term, and rebuild damaged and injured tissue.

Tissue damage like an ACL tear or having ACL reconstruction has three stages of healing processes; inflammation, proliferation, and remodeling. During the inflammation stage your body draws healing chemicals to the injured area which usually causes pain, swelling, redness, and heat to the area. The inflammation stage usually occurs for the first few days or week after your ACL tear and for the first week to two weeks after your ACL surgery.

During this time it can help to eat more anti-inflammatory fats like olive oil, avocados, fish oil, flax oil or ground flax, including fish, like salmon or sardines, and mixed nuts or seeds. Include inflammation managing herbs and spices like turmeric (7 tsp/day), garlic (2-4 cloves/day or 600-1200mg garlic extract), and bromelain from pineapple (2 cups pineapple/day or bromelain capsules). Other foods like cocoa, tea, and berries are also beneficial during the inflammation stage of healing because the antioxidants and anti-inflammatory properties provide support to your body when healing the injured area and help to control excess inflammation.

The proliferation and remodeling stages are somewhat similar. During the proliferation stage damaged tissues are removed via the circulatory system and new blood supply and temporary tissue is built to set up the healing process. Without a successful inflammation stage the body wouldn't be ready to remove the damaged tissues. The remodeling stage is the final stage and is a more long-term healing stage. During the remodeling stage stronger, more permanent tissues replace the temporary tissue. During this stage the tunnels in your femur and tibia drilled to hold your ACL will start to remodel and heal, and the ACL itself will begin to bind to your tissue and create new cells and collagen to return it to normal function.

During the second and third stages energy intake is top priority. If you aren't providing your body with a sufficient amount of food, then it will not have enough energy to properly heal all of these tissues. This stage doesn't have any fancy requirements other than maintaining your energy levels by eating a mixed variety of fruits, vegetables, healthy fats, carbohydrates, and lean proteins. The same healthy eating principles apply avoiding processed foods, sugar, and artificial dyes and chemicals. Food is fuel.

Below are a few vitamins and minerals that will aid your restorative process during all three stages of healing. Remember it is best to get all of your nutrients through real healthy food instead of supplements and processed food sources; although an occasional supplement is okay if you feel you are lacking in any of these nutrients. If you are eating a nutrient dense, varied, and balanced diet then you should be consuming most of these through food alone. These vitamins and minerals have many distinct properties that are very beneficial for the body but specifically applying them towards your ACL repair is the main goal of this chapter.

7.2.1 Vitamin A

Vitamin A speeds up the production of collagen which is a vital protein in your ACL. As you might recall in Chapter 3.1.3, estrogen can have an effect in decreasing the collagen production of the ACL causing some women to have a greater incidence of injury than others. Vitamin A will not totally cure those symptoms but it will have an effect on the collagen production and for women with higher estrogen levels, usually during childbearing years and during puberty, this can help to increase collagen production for your ACL but it will not totally eliminate estrogen's effects.

Vitamin A can be found in a large variety of foods including sweet potatoes, carrots, kale, squash, romaine lettuce, prunes, dried apricots, cantaloupe, melon, red pepper, mango, and blue fin tuna.

7.2.2 Vitamin C

When you consume Vitamin C and Vitamin E, they work together to decrease inflammation and increase strength. Not only immune system strength but strength rebuilding after surgery can be increased from ingesting adequate levels of Vitamin C and E along with your healthy diet and rehabilitation program. Vitamin C can be found in foods like fruits and vegetables, specifically broccoli, bell peppers, cauliflower, strawberries, and berries.

7.2.3 Vitamin E

Vitamin E helps to minimize oxidative stress and inflammation of your knee after surgery which allows for greater strength gains and a faster recovery process. Vitamin E can be found in spinach, almonds, roasted sun flower seeds, avocados, fish, broccoli, and olive oils. Note,

Vitamin E has a special role in anti-inflammatory effects which is why so many Vitamin E rich foods are recommended during the inflammation stage of healing. Similar to putting Vitamin E on sunburn, ingesting foods high in Vitamin E can have the same healing effects inside your body.

7.2.4 Flavonoids

Flavonoids help to reduce swelling by protecting cells from oxygen damage, blood vessels from rupture or leakage, and by enhancing the power of your Vitamin C absorption. This is important because of the high risk of blood clots during and after surgery and the sedentary nature of your recovery decreasing the amount of blood flow through your vessels. Foods high in flavonoids are apples, blueberries, strawberries, tomatoes, onions, cabbage, and black beans.

7.2.5 Zinc

Zinc helps to maintain a strong immune system similar to that of Vitamin C. This is always very important when recovering from surgery. Any infection to your body will decrease the chances of healing from your procedure because the body will have more work to do to eliminate the virus or infection causing it to decrease its healing power after your surgery. Zinc can be found in foods like seafood, spinach, chia seeds, flax seeds, nuts especially almonds and pecans, and chicken.

Ask the Expert: *Linda Citron, Board Certified Health and Nutrition Coach, citronnutrition.com*

"I highly recommend discussing your diet and nutritional

needs with your doctor and/or surgeon, because specific surgeries may require medically-approved, pre- and post-surgery dietary adjustments. Make sure you let your doctor know of any medications you take on a daily basis, and the amount of alcohol you consume, as that may be an influencing factor in your surgery and recovery.

My number one piece of advice is to get your body and immune system in the best shape you can prior to surgery to improve the speed of your recovery, and you want to sustain healthy eating post-surgery to help with the speed of healing. Since we're on the subject of sugar, reducing or eliminating sugar and highly-processed foods prior to and following surgery will help your body recover and heal and will reduce the impact sugar could have on post-surgery inflammation and joint pain. I also recommend "crowding out" processed and refined foods with nutrient-dense whole foods, including green vegetables, vegetable-based soups, lean protein such as fish, and healthy fats, such as olive oil, almonds and avocados, to name a few.

I also think it is important to consistently drink water to ensure you are well hydrated prior to surgery, and also post-surgery, to help your body detoxify itself of foreign substances such as anesthesia. A good rule of thumb for every day is to drink half your weight in ounces of water each day. For example, if you weigh 140 pounds, you would drink at minimum 70 ounces of water every day. For post-surgery, I would recommend adding freshly squeezed lemon into your morning water (if your doctor approves), which acts as a detoxifying agent."

KEY POINTS

- Losing excess weight and body fat before surgery will help to decrease surgical health related complications and will aid in your recovery process on crutches and as you progress into strength training.
- Eating nutrient dense and varied diet rich in vitamins and minerals is key to having a happy, healthy body. During recovery from ACL surgery the nutrients you eat and drink will either enhance or slow down your progress.
- Drink lots of water pre and post-operative besides when they limit you the evening before your surgery.
- You are what you eat!

8

SLEEP

Sleep is a huge part of being healthy that often gets overlooked. We spend nearly one third of our lives asleep. Our body requires sleep as a basic function just like it does water and food. Sleep is an important aspect of healing not to be taken lightly. On a normal night, it is best to get a minimum of eight hours of sleep, although most Americans do not reach that amount on a regular basis. While recovering from surgery it can be difficult to fall asleep because of pain levels, anxiety from surgery and pain, and being uncomfortable. Although it would be nice to take your recovery time and binge watch your favorite guilty pleasures on Netflix, this view point will not help you to recover.

Sleep is a natural state of rest required by our bodies every day in order to rebuild, repair, rejuvenate, and recover. Normally it is essential to recover yourself from your day to day life functions but after surgery sleep is even more integral because your body is working overtime to heal you. If you do not allow yourself the proper rest during your recovery, your body is going to be working even harder then it needs to. This goes from the first day out of surgery until months after your procedure.

Try practicing better sleep habits even before your surgery. This will aid your efforts when you have pain and discomfort effecting your sleep cycle. Make sure to set aside at least eight hours for you to sleep and shut off all electronics and lights one hour before bedtime. Without the proper amount of darkness the body cannot take on a relaxed state and it will be harder for you to fall asleep. The hour of darkness before bed is a wonderful time to practice your mindful meditation. It is also a mindful sleep practice to avoid late night snacking. Try to make sure that your last meal is at least two hours before your quiet hour. We do not need the digestive system keeping you awake or messing up your relaxation. Turn on a fan or some peaceful nature sounds to block out any outside noise or distractions in your household or your neighborhood. Stay silent and focus on your breathing. Breathe in deeply through the diaphragm and breathe out slowly. Think about your positive affirmations: "I can, I will, I am." Or, think about absolutely nothing. This is a peaceful state so make sure you do not allow any negative or anxious thoughts or energy into existence. If you have trouble thinking of nothing, then focus on something that makes you happy or repeat your positive affirmations to ensure that no negativity is allowed to surface itself.

After your surgery, sleep might be more difficult. But, by establishing these healthy sleep practices hopefully your body will be used to the relaxation triggers and it will help you to fall asleep easier. During your weeks at home recovering try to get as much sleep as possible. Your body is in survival mode trying to heal you and sleep is going to make that process happen even faster. Aim for nine or ten hours of sleep the week after your surgery and make it a goal for yourself to get a minimum of eight hours of sleep every night during all of your recovery months. Even when you think you have healed, your body will be continually experiencing trauma as you work hard to gain back range of motion and strength at your muscles. You are starting over from scratch so it's going to be a difficult process but sleep is your friend.

Chapter Recap

- Sleep is a key part of the recovery process. From the day after your surgery all the way to six months out of your surgery, your body is going to be fighting to recover, gain strength, and relearn skills which will use up a lot of energy.
- Set a new sleep schedule allowing yourself 1 full hour of dark, quiet time before bedtime and a minimum of eight hours for actual sleep time.

9

ACL REHABILITATION

The statistics for athletes returning to the same level of play as before their ACL surgery are good but not great. "Even in high level with published data, the return to play rate (meaning you play at least one snap in the NFL) is somewhere around 63%, which means that 27% of these athletes never play another down in the NFL. They blow their ACL and they never come back. These are supremely conditioned athletes with the best physical therapists and the best trainers with the best rehab and genetically they are specimens and for 27% of them it's a career ending injury"-Dr. Tom Myers. Many athletes do not return to playing sports due to re-injury, weakness, being scared or needing revision surgery. I haven't played sports since I was 14-years-old, when I tore my ACL for the second time. After that, improper placement of the ACL in my surgery and failed cadaver grafts caused me to end up needing revision surgeries. It is very rare to have only one ACL injury and my mission is to change these statistics. Regardless there are many factors that go into a successful recovery process and not all athletes return to the level they were at before injury unlike some of the pro athletes who make it seem like a commonplace task. That being said, we see athletes make the amazing comeback all the time but we also shouldn't expect the comeback to be as easy as it is for our favorite professional athletes. Remember they have highly renowned strength coaches, physical therapists, orthopedic surgeons, and athletic trainers at their disposal every day through their recovery, and their recovery is their full-time job.

One level of concern regarding ACL rehabilitation is the limitation of insurance on physical therapy visits. A progressive and complete ACL rehabilitation program should return you to the same level of activity as before the injury without any compensations. But, when patients are limited to 20 or 30 post-op visits they are not receiving the highest quality of care and worse, some patients are under the impression that when their insurance visits run out they are fully recovered. Normally this is a skewed viewpoint and one that can cause your knee dramatic long term damage.

"Modern day surgery is so advanced that patients get their range of motion back and start moving without a limp or pain so quick some of the patients want to quit therapy too soon. This issue is that the patient thinks they are so indestructible so fast that they don't understand the entire process of the rehabilitation from a neuroscience standpoint or from a regular exercise standpoint. It bothers me because when we got introduced to manage care 20-

something years ago we started getting limited visits for insurance companies and now it's a very big challenge for us clinicians to be able to take those limited visits and stretch them out in order to create a good 3-phase rehabilitation program for the patient in order to reach their functional goals. Limited visits challenge us because patients want to quit too quick either because they feel like they can or they run out of visits or run out of money" *Terry Trundle ATC LAT PTA.*

If you want to return to the level of play you had before surgery, you need to approach your recovery with the mindset of a professional athlete. You will need to find a support system and you will need to work on your rehabilitation every single day. Make sure that you find a physical therapist who will evaluate you as an individual and not just a textbook ACL rehab patient. Make sure that you are ready to hire your physical therapist out-of-pocket after insurance runs out or hire another Exercise Professional when your physical therapy insurance runs out. This book will help you to avoid extra out-of-pocket costs, but remember, it is extremely beneficial to have a knowledgeable expert supervising your rehabilitation if at all possible.

Take your rehabilitation seriously. You and you alone have the power and resources to make the ultimate comeback but your success is all dependent on your approach, attitude, and dedication to your recovery and rehabilitation. It will take daily work. This could possibly be one of the hardest things that you ever do, but it is well worth it because it will determine the long-term mobility, stability, and longevity of your knee. Not only does your injured knee have a huge incidence of re-injury but so does your non-surgical knee. These are the only knees you have and it is essential to protect them.

The following section includes samples and tips for your rehabilitation journey. You will be working with an experienced physical therapist but I wanted to include some extra guidance for your off days and my expert recommendations for mastering each phase of rehabilitation. These are the signature moves that Terry Trundle has mentored with me for the past 12 years. He is the "knee man" and has taught me everything I know. Your rehabilitation program will consist of many other exercises that are extremely beneficial as well but through my many experiences with ACL recovery I recommend mastering all of these exercises before progressing in your rehabilitation. These are meant for you to do at home or at your local gym in addition or conjunction with your physical therapy visits. These are not prescribed rehabilitation or customized moves for your body so seeking a specialist to work with you one on one is preferred.

9.1 FIRST TWO WEEKS!

For the first two to four weeks after your surgery the biggest areas of focus are resting, decreasing swelling, gaining range of motion, and regaining muscle control. As mentioned before, swelling is the main focus during the first two weeks of recovery because less swelling means less muscle weakness. Increases in swelling after surgery are associated with atrophy or weakness in the muscles and decreased range of motion which can both extremely hinder your progress and cause potential long-term damage. "Arthrofibrosis, which is internal scarring, is one of the biggest issues with ACL surgery. That means the patient doesn't get off to a good start with motion, has excessive swelling, demonstrates a high level of pain, and just doesn't do the right things"-*Terry Trundle ATC LAT PTA*. Do not try to be the hero and overdo your activity because swelling is a big deal and can detrimentally halt or hinder your recovery. That is why it is so essential to do everything that you can to put your life on hold for two weeks of quality recovery time after your surgery. Of course this is not an easy task, but it will benefit you in the long run if you can make it work. By following my tips and tricks for managing the first two weeks you will be off to a great start on your goals.

9.1.1 DECREASE SWELLING

As mentioned in Section 5.1, swelling is the biggest concern coming out of your surgery. It is important to keep pain management in control and muscle atrophy at a minimum and will help you to gain more range of motion faster because it will allow for fewer restrictions in your physical therapy. After ACL surgery, you can't ice too much. Follow the protocol listed in the chart in Section 9.1.3 on how long to keep ice on the knee and how long to let the knee thaw out. Many athletes make the mistake of leaving ice constantly on the knee but if you do not allow proper blood flow back to the area, the ice treatment will have less effect. I recommend following the chart for the first four to seven days after surgery to ensure that you are staying on top of your swelling and pain. It will also be very painful to remove your leg from an elevated position and bring it below heart level in order to go to the restroom. Follow the chart for an easy way to allow blood flow to slowly return to the knee before crutching yourself to the restroom.

If you overdo it and have a swelling mishap, elevate the knee on your foam wedge and work on ABC circles. Literally write out the alphabet using your foot and ankle. Try to get as much movement and range of motion as you can without causing any pain to your knee. This will serve two purposes; it will push excess swelling out of the foot by increasing blood flow to the area and getting it moving along the circulatory system and it also works well when you elevate your foot for too long and lose blood flow. Make sure to always keep good blood flow through the foot. This is why it is important to follow the elevation and ice chart in Section 9.1.3.

Tip! Try my favorite anti-inflammatory drink. This will help to hydrate you, detox your system from anesthesia drugs, and aid in your inflammatory systems post-op as well as aid in digestion which is much needed following major surgery. Take 20 ounces of water and heat up to warmer than room temperature. Add in ½ of a lemon, 1 teaspoon of turmeric, 1 teaspoon of ginger, 1 pinch of cinnamon, and 2-4 tablespoons of apple cider vinegar. The apple cider vinegar will make it taste a little sour, so decrease that amount if you don't like the taste, but as you get used to the drink it will begin to taste better. This is my morning staple! I notice a difference in pain levels on the days that I don't drink my anti-inflammatory drink.

9.1.2 GAINING RANGE OF MOTION

Gaining range of motion is going to come from the decrease in swelling but also through hard work. Gaining flexion at the knee or bending is very important for recovery and rehabilitation, for the most important portion of your initial therapy is going to be regaining full extension and being able to fully straighten your knee. "Full extension of the knee is so important in order to facilitate leg control that leads in to normal ambulation, no pain and no swelling" *Terry Trundle ATC LAT PTA*. Full extension can help to avoid surgery complications like arthrofibrosis.

A CPM Machine is great to use after surgery, as permitted by your surgeon. The CPM machine can be set to a certain degree of flexion (bend) and a certain degree of extension (straighten) for the knee based on the restrictions set by your surgeon or physical therapist. It is important to use the CPM machine because it involuntarily moves your leg which helps to keep blow flow to the area and helps to gain range of motion and keep you from getting very stiff. Many patients are in so much pain that they avoid moving the knee which, long term, makes it more painful and can leave you stuck in a position with very decreased range of motion.

If the CPM machine is not recommended for you then you can still do some stretches that will ensure you don't tighten up. The half-moon stretch (described below) is a great way to gain extension (straightening) at the knee. This might cause you to tighten up a little, which is okay, so it is also good to perform hamstring co-contractions in conjunction with the half-moon hamstring stretch. The half-moon hamstrings stretch a similar set up to the hamstring co-contractions. Sit upright on a firm bed or table and allow your heel to hang slightly off of the edge of the bed or table. Make sure you extend your knee by pushing your heel forward and bringing your knee to a straightened or extended position. Keeping your spine straight, lean forward at the hips until you feel a comfortable stretch at the hamstrings. Hold for 30 to 60 seconds while breathing deeply through the diaphragm. This would be best performed before using the restroom to allow slow and gradual blood flow to the leg after elevating it or after you perform your hamstring co-contractions (described in next section.)

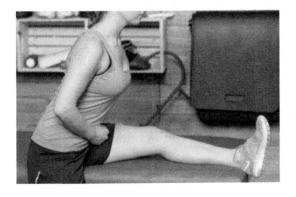

Towel slides are a great way to work on knee flexion (bending.) To begin, sit down on the floor or on your bed, and make sure the surface is flat. Use a towel or a dog leash to wrap around your foot gently. Make sure you have a small washcloth underneath your foot or a sock on so that it is able to slide. Now gently and slowly pull on the towel or dog leash to slide your foot towards you bending your knee as much as you are able to. Do not force the move, only do what feels comfortable. When you can't get any more motion, slowly release the tension and ease your leg back to the straightened position. Again, most surgeons and physical therapists will tell you what degree of flexion or bending you are allowed to do as well as what degree of extension or straightening of the knee they will allow based on your procedure or limitations. Perform anywhere from 10 to 15 reps and 3 or 4 sets per day based on strength and pain. Be cautious and don't overdo the move. These exercises or the CPM machine should be done every single day, pain permitted, until you have full range of motion back.

Another great trick is using a muscle stick self-massage roller (mentioned in surgery prep list.) These are easy to buy online and will provide you with relief when your leg muscles get tight from surgery and recovery. It is much easier to use than a foam roller when injured but applies the same basic principles. Self-massage is a way to decrease tension at muscles. By rolling up and down along the belly of the muscle and applying firm resistance your muscles will stay loose. Surgery and injury can make them overly tight due to compensations and pain. Make sure that you don't roll over a joint, only the muscles. But this technique can give you great relief in your quads, hamstrings, and calves while you are unable to do a ton of stretches or foam rolling.

9.1.3 REGAINING MUSCLE CONTROL

As your pain starts to decrease, it is time to start addressing those muscles. As mentioned previously, the muscle weakness in your leg is going to be significant and even doing small exercises can help aid in your recovery process. After surgery, the neuromuscular connection between the brain and the muscles can be delayed or even difficult to initiate. This is your body's response to pain and trauma in order to help you rest and heal, but the longer you go without activating these muscles the harder it can be to get them to regain function. Using an electrical stimulation unit can help you to reactivate the muscles weakened and shut down after surgery. Electrical stimulation sometimes referred to as "e-stem" or TENS is a recovery technique that can be used in two ways; to relieve pain or to re-educate muscles. The devices come in many different sizes and usually have two basic settings; high frequency and low frequency. Low frequency settings are used for muscle re-education and create a constant pulsing involuntary contraction at the muscles. With inactivity, injury, surgery or even stroke, patients can lose control and firing capacity at certain muscle groups. It is the body's defense mechanism against pain. By applying the pads onto the muscle belly and using the machine to passively contract the muscles, a patient can get the muscle re-firing with more ease. It is best to use active techniques (like the hamstring co contractions and quad set pluses detailed next) to teach the patient to fire their muscle simultaneously with the help of the machine in order to re-learn the muscle firing capabilities and re-teach the neuromuscular system to activate that muscle on its own.

In untrained individuals or in those rehabilitating from injury, electrical stimulation has been shown to be more effective than voluntary activations in eliciting beneficial gains. Research has shown that only 71% of the muscle tissue is activated during maximal efforts in untrained or injured populations. When the ability to maximally recruit motor units is limited with injury or being untrained, it affects your mechanics in turn leading to pain and injury. It's a perpetual cycle which is why it is so important to eliminate muscle imbalances before returning to sport.

High frequency settings create a constant buzzing providing pain relief to the muscle or joint. In theory, this works pretty simply. Pain signals are sent to the brain via nerves. The stimulation sensation for electrical stimulation on high frequency settings is said to block the nerves that deliver these signals.

It is ideal to activate the hamstrings first as you begin simple rehabilitation because for one, activation of the quads with quad sets or straight leg raises will more than likely cause a lot of unnecessary pain because it compresses the knee while it is already in a lot of pain. It will also further reinforce the improper sequencing involved in quad dominance which for a female athlete it can be extremely beneficial to focus on hamstring co contractions after surgery in order to change the natural sequencing of their body. Hamstring exercises help to decompress the knee which decreases pain. Quad sets are an extremely beneficial way to build back your quad muscles after surgery and the quads are very important to strengthen after surgery but it would be best to hold off on those until your pain is manageable and your hamstrings are firing flawlessly.

"My biggest emphasis is co contractions; hamstrings over

quad contractions. The modern terminology for co contraction is co-activation and if you looked into the modern literature that is published in ACL rehabilitation literature what you will find is co activation influence. Get the hamstrings to fire faster, get the hamstrings to fire quicker before the quads, and therefore I teach this principle: Improperly performed quad set exercises compresses the knee because it's painful and it's swollen. To decompress the knee, you create a hamstring isometric contraction and allow the quadriceps muscles to be activated in the secondary state and you get a decompression. This creates a leg control activity that is going to decrease their pain. It has been shown in the research literature that hamstrings can decompress the pain in the knee while the quadriceps muscles are being retrained" *Terry Trundle ACT LAT PTA.*

Tip! In many physical therapy programs a very commonly prescribed exercise is the straight leg raise. Straight leg raises are a very outdated approach to ACL rehabilitation and Terry Trundle has disproved its benefits in recent years at his lecture seminars. "From a strengthening standpoint in the first phase of rehab is core strength and core stabilization; this is important, but the key to post-op ACL rehabilitation is the core becomes the hip. The hip strength particularly in abduction motion, extension, and rotation is very important. I de-emphasize performing straight leg raises as a rehabilitation exercise because they have very little value from a standpoint of therapeutic value based on the evidence of the exercise. What happens is the straight leg raise becomes a test for the patient to have leg control but it doesn't have anything to do with the recovery of the quadriceps muscle or anything of the surrounding muscles. But when you think about lateral leg raises and standing leg raises on the cable machine and standing mini squats, the things that create interaction of the hip to the knee through the foot being stabilized are really important. That is why the early use of closed chain exercises is so important" *Terry Trundle ATC LAT PTA.*

Straight leg raises are also usually painful for many post-op patients which is why decompressing the knee with hamstring co-contractions listed below are the best approach. By strengthening the muscles of the quads with closed chain exercises like the ones listed in Section 9.2, the athlete will regain better control and function at the knee. Remember everything in the body is connected and influences the muscles and joints above it and below. Straight leg raises have no value to the strength or stability at the hip which will not add therapeutic value to your rehabilitation program as the hip and glute muscles are critical in the function of the knee. In addition to not including the hip, the straight leg raise gives the patient no contact with the foot on the ground. So why are we preforming our rehabilitation without involving the foot and hip? In Section 9.2, you will learn some great strengthening exercises that include the foot and hip.

To activate the hamstrings safely, sit upright on a firm bed, table, or the floor. Straighten your leg as best as you can by pushing your heel forward. Take one hand and place it on the bottom of your thigh grasping your hamstrings muscles. Squeeze and contract the hamstrings into your hand and hold for five seconds. You might have a little bit of quad activation and that is okay but make sure that you are contracting and activation your hamstrings primarily. Start out with 3 sets of 12 reps once or twice per day and if you have no pain you can slowly advance your numbers each day. Try 4 sets of 12 and then 3 sets of 15. Try repeating these exercises multiple times per day to ensure that you are getting activation at the hamstrings readily.

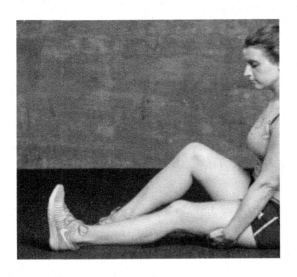

After 9 to 15 days when your pain is dwindling, it is okay to add in quad set pluses. Remember that is best to hold off on quad set pluses until you can perform them without pain. The timing might be different for each patient. Quad set pluses are very similar to the hamstring co-contraction but remember activating the hamstrings first can help with many athletes, practically female athletes, who experience quad dominance. The idea is to teach the brain to fire the hamstrings before the quads ideally allowing a less chance of knee injury because the hamstrings are one of the major muscle groups protecting the knee.

To start your quad set plus, sit upright on a flat table or bed. Straighten your leg with your heel down on the table. Notice, there will be a natural gap between your knee and the table. Now squeeze and contract your quads once, hold, and then squeeze it a second time allowing the VMO muscle (small muscle in the quads located on the inside of the leg just above the kneecap) to finally contract. Hold for a few seconds and then release. Repeat 15 -20 times as long as there is no pain. Work your way up from 2 sets to 3,4, and 5. The photo on the left is the start position and the right is the position of the quad set that you hold.

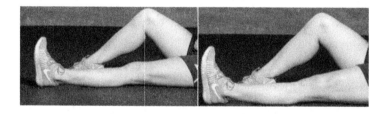

Here's an example of a balanced routine to keep your muscles stimulated, pain levels down, and swelling at a minimum. Repeat this all hours you are awake if possible. Take note the technique for slowly allowing blood flow to return to the knee very gradually. If you are elevating your knee and quickly bring it down below heart level to crutch to the bathroom, the sudden rush of blood flow is going to be very painful. Make sure you gradually bring the knee below heart level and even perform your exercises to get some healthy blood circulation steadily versus all at once before you need to move yourself.

12pm Ice and elevate knee above heart level	2:30pm Slowly transition your leg from elevated to lower position
12:20pm Remove Ice, continue to elevate	2:35pm Begin hamstring co contractions and quad set pluses once blood flow has circulated back into knee
1pm Slowly transition your leg from elevated to a lower position while you are seated on the bed or couch. Gradual. Only a few inches at a time and then allow blood flow to slowly go to your knee.	2:50pm Complete exercises and crutch to the bathroom if needed while blood flow is at knee
1:05pm Begin Hamstring co contractions and quad set pluses once blood flow has circulated back into the knee gradually	Repeat all day long. If you get tired or have increased pain then you can skip your exercises for an hour or two but use the same time schedule for ice, removing ice, and allowing blood flow back to your knee before you move around.
1:20pm Complete exercises and crutch to the restroom while blood flow is at the knee	20 minutes of ice followed by 40 minutes to let the knee thaw out. Repeat.
1:30pm Ice and elevate knee	
1:50pm Remove Ice, continue to elevate	

9.2 RETURN TO FUNCTION

By now you're getting past the first week or two after surgery. It is grueling, boring, and more importantly, it's very tedious. All of these little exercises might seem pointless or mundane but they are of great importance to not only your surgical knee but to your good knee too. After tearing your ACL, you have a 1 in 50 chance of tearing it again on either knee. These are huge odds and it is so important to address the biomechanics of your body's compensations now in order to incorporate corrective exercise into your rehabilitation for both knees. Even if you feel that you are walking normal and able to do a simple workout without restriction you are most likely wrong. Even the slightest change in your biomechanics can alter your movement patterns causing you to be more prone to injury.

The goals during this phase of rehabilitation are increasing quadriceps, hamstrings, and abductor strength, increasing balance and proprioceptive awareness, increasing endurance, and increasing core and glutes strength. At a certain point in your rehabilitation journey it is going to be crucial to preform your rehab exercises on both legs. Some of the exercises might feel easy on your uninjured leg and that is okay, but any weaknesses or compensations that you have in that leg can be addressed at the same time. You will be integrating squats and other two-legged exercises during this phase and it is important to be working with a professional that can look at the entire body as a whole to ensure that you aren't compensating on one leg as you begin to retrain your body into squats, deadlifts, lunges, and step ups.

Each leg will alter the other leg so both leg knees to be addressed. Of course, one leg will be significantly weaker than the other and this will take a lot of hard work to catch up, but it is integral that you don't begin any intense weight bearing exercises like long distance running or sports until your strength is equal on both legs.

This can end up causing compensations and ultimately give you pain in your good leg, your back, or your hips. Some of this is going to happen anyway just because of the strength difference in each leg, but we don't want to over promote this tendency by going on long runs or doing too much.

With limitations regarding insurance, many ACL rehabilitation journeys are cut short. This is terrible and do not let insurance impede your progress! There are many out-of-pocket specialists that are highly qualified to guide you through the entirety of your rehabilitation process.

9.2.1 INCREASING HAMSTRINGS, QUADRICEPS, AND ABDUCTOR STRENGTH

Gaining strength is going to be difficult at first. The light weight easy exercises are going to be tiring and mundane but remember they serve an important focus. By regaining strength and learning to fire the muscles again it will allow us to get a head start on decreasing your injury rate on both of your knees.

Hamstrings- The hamstrings are much more resilient than the quads and typically are a little easier to strength following ACL surgery. More importantly, we want to reinforce the firing patterns of the hamstrings first following ACL surgery, especially in the female athlete because most female athletes are quad dominant, refer to Chapter 3.1 for more information.

Remember how you perform your hamstring co-contractions before you did your quad sets? It's the same idea here. The hamstrings control eccentric motions at the knee and help you to decelerate safely when changing directions or sprinting. A lag in time of the firing sequence in the hamstrings can lead to injury. Right now we are just working on basic strength and range of motion, but later these actions will be incorporated functionally in your rehabilitation to ensure a proper recovery.

Exercises are listed in order of difficulty. Do not advance yourself to the next exercise until you have mastered Exercise 1 without any pain.

Exercise 1: Single Leg Hamstring Curl – *on machine or with band*

If using a band, begin sitting on the edge of a table with a band around your ankle and someone holding it at a 30-degree angle with as much resistance as you can tolerate without pain. Start at the top of the movement and slowly bend the knee driving the heel inward creating force on the band with the hamstrings. Perform to full-range-of-motion and very slowly in both directions on the way in and the way out. Keep resistance on the band the entire time.

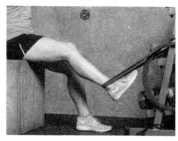 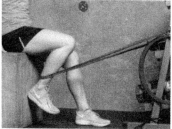

If using a hamstring curl machine, place your leg in the machine with a natural angle from the hip. Try to keep the foot somewhat even with how wide your hip is. Push the heel down driving your leg in and your knee to bend while activating the hamstrings. Bring to full-range-of-motion and keep control in both directions of the movement.

Exercise 2: Standing Cable Extension

Begin facing the cable machine with the working leg secured. Activate your quads slightly (similar to your quad set plus) and slightly squeeze your glutes. While holding these small activations and keeping your leg straight (but not hyperextended) bring your leg straight back about 3 to 8 inches. Keep control of the movement and slowly bring your leg back into the starting position.

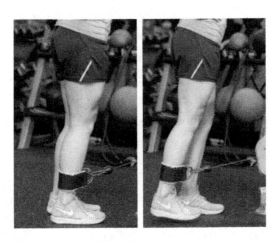

Exercise 3: Hamstring Curls on Stability Ball

Lay down on the floor on your back with your feet spaced hip width apart on top of a stability ball. Begin by bridging your hips up into the air as your starting position. Pull your feet inwards by bending the knees and driving the hips up into the air. You should be pulling with your hamstrings but also keep your glutes and core involved in the move. Slowly lower your hips and straighten your knees to return to the starting position.

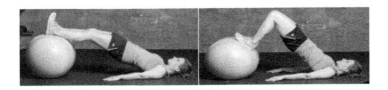

Quads - Remember, the function of the quadriceps is huge in control and stability at the knee but we want to make sure that we are gaining back control of the VMO in the quads. After ACL surgery it can be even harder to fire the VMO muscle located on the inside of your quads down near the knee cap. This is the same muscle that you were trying to activate in the quad set pluses during Section 9.1.3. The lateral or outside of your quads should have a much easier time firing and gaining strength after surgery but we need to be careful not to let that muscle take over because it can cause problems in the future.

Exercise 1: Terminal Knee Extension or TKE's

Begin standing using a resistance band around the back of the knee that has enough resistance for your strength level. The working leg will have the band around the knee and the non-working leg will be half a foot length behind the working leg foot. Start with a slight bend in the working leg and little to no resistance on the band. Contract the quads, most importantly the VMO on the inside of the quad, to pull the band backward and straighten the knee. Keep tension on the band and return to the beginning position.

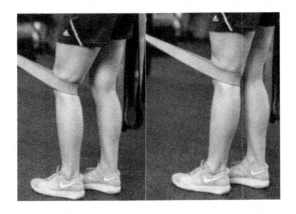

Exercise 2: Standing Cable Flexion

Begin facing away from the cable machine with your working leg secured. Slightly squeeze your quad and glutes and while keeping your leg straight (but not hyperextended) bring your leg forward about 3 to 5 inches using your quads. Slowly bring the leg back to the starting positions keeping tension on the move.

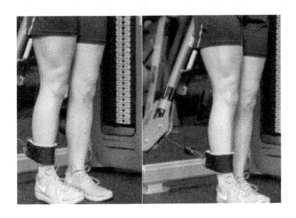

Exercise 3: Eccentric VMO Step Down

Using a small step (anywhere from 3 inches to 6 inches); stand with the working leg even and level on the step and slowly lower yourself to the floor with the heel of the non-working leg as first and only contact to the floor.

Do not rest, simply tap the floor and slowly bring yourself back to the starting point.

Keep your hips back with the weight in your glutes and do not allow your knee to come in front of your toe. You should feel this move in your VMO located on the inside of your quads. Final position pictured.

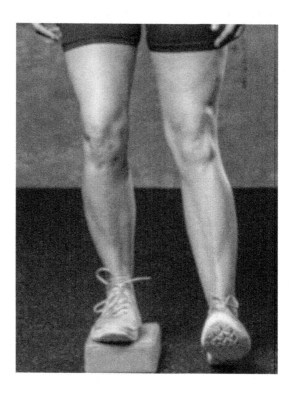

Exercise 4: Step Up to Balance

Put one foot on the top of the box and step onto the box driving your opposite leg into the air. Do not allow your knee to go in front of your toe. Make sure you are using your quads and your glutes in this move. Step all the way back down onto the floor and repeat.

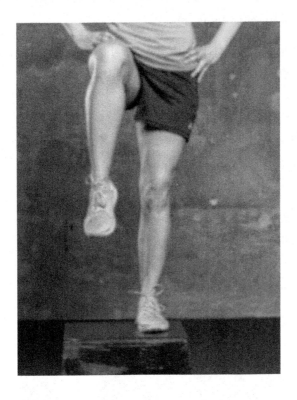

Exercise 5: Modified Single Leg Ball Wall Squat or Single Leg TRX squat

Place the ball against the wall and on the small of your back. Bring both legs far in front of your hips so that you have a good angle to start your squat. Remove one leg and either hold it in the air or put it behind you for a little bit or balance/strength support. Slowly lower down into a single leg squat position keeping your knee behind your toes and return to the start position.

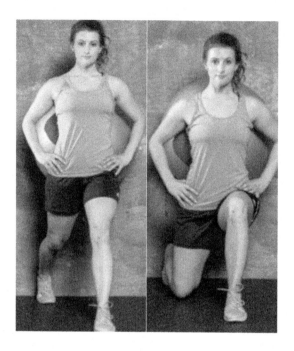

Tip! - Try RNT if you are having trouble with avoiding knee valgus in this move. This is common for those with a wider Q angle and those who suffer from chronic VMO weakness.

Reactive Neuromuscular Training or RNT uses outside resistance to neurologically turn on an automatic response. It teaches the muscles and the brain to resist and react to the applied force on the band allowing the body to recruit muscles that have weakened and become inefficient over time. RNT helps to increase neuromuscular coordination and improve joint stability which are both two common issues regarding ACL rehabilitation.

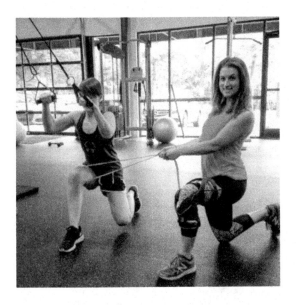

The example in the picture is my client Kim. She has had four knee surgeries on her right knee and suffers from chronic instability and knee valgus due to weakness and chronic VMO issues resulting from her surgeries. By using the resistance band in the direction of her compensation problem at the VMO muscle (located on the lower quad on the inside), her brain and muscles are forced to resist the force on the band and in turn will relearn proper firing sequence patterns that will eventually help decrease her knee pain and prevent her from suffering further knee injuries. This is huge from someone who has had this many procedures and is unable to fire and coordinate the proper muscle actions efficiently without the band. Kim teaches five Bootcamp classes every week and is already seeing tremendous results on her rehab allowing her to instruct and teach her Bootcamp with no pain and no dysfunction!

Exercise 6: Side Lunge

Start with your legs wider than hip width apart. Lunge down to one side keeping your hips and butt back like you were sitting one cheek onto a bench. Keep your hips directly over your foot and knee. Return to starting position.

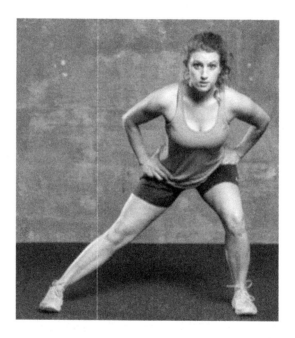

Abductors – The abductors of your legs and hips are the muscles that control actions where your leg is moving away from your body. Our main focus in this phase of rehab is your gluteus medius muscle. This muscle is very important for the functioning of your knee and leg but more importantly a strong gluteus medius can help decrease the effects of knee valgus, and over pronation at the foot. These are anatomical variations that if not fixed will continue to contribute to knee strain or further injury in the future.

Exercise 1: Standing Cable Abduction

Begin facing the working leg farthest away from the cable machine with it secured to the machine. Straighten your knee, slightly squeezing your quad and glutes and pull your leg away from the resistance about 3 to 5 inches. You should be pulling your leg away from your body slowly and then bring it back to the start position. Keeping tension on the muscle slowly bring your leg back to the start position.

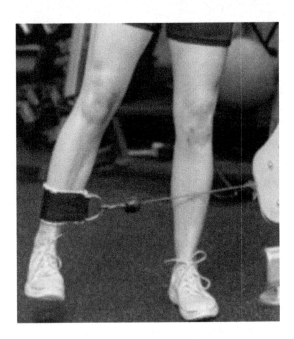

Exercise 2: Lateral Tube Walking

Use a band with enough resistance for your strength level. Place the band around both legs slightly above the knees. Keep constant tension on the band so start with your legs hip width apart where you feel tension and take a small step to the side; stepping with each foot. Continue on for 12 to 15 steps and then return to the starting point by performing 12 to 15 reps coming back with the other leg leading.

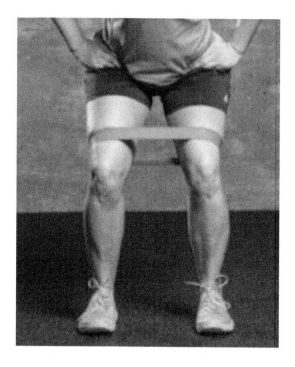

Exercise 3: Lateral Step up to Balance

Begin facing to the side of the step. With the leg closest to the step, step up onto the platform and drive your opposite leg into the air. Make sure that your knee stays behind your toe. Return back to the start position.

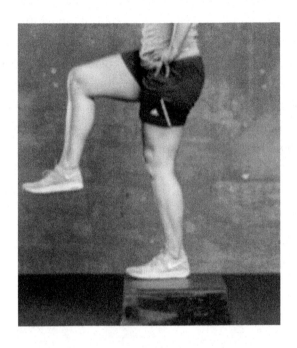

9.2.2 INCREASING BALANCE AND PROPRIOCEPTIVE AWARENESS

After injury or surgery, the receptors in your muscles, tendons, and ligaments can lose their efficiency. These receptors communicate with your brain and spinal cord to let your body know where it is in space so that it can produce complex and integral movements. Remember that the ACL is a mechanoreceptor meaning that it also sends messages to the brain and spinal cord regarding positioning, spacial awareness, and reaction time. Because of these reasons balance training is a huge part of your rehabilitation program. Obviously you need to increase the strength in your stabilizer muscles (the muscles recruited for balance, stability, and posture) in order to advance to harder training but after your balance and stability returns incorporating reaction training can help the ACL and other mechanoreceptors damaged in your injury and surgery to repair and replenish their firing capabilities.

When beginning balance training it is important to remember that the body is a kinetic chain and that everything works together. The muscles on the bottom of your foot relate and communicate with the muscles in your pelvic floor. These muscles work together to stabilize your body in many different ways. When preforming these balance exercises make sure that your foot is flat on the ground and you are slightly gripping with all of your toes with your heel on the ground. It is great to practice your balance training bare foot as it allows all of the muscles in your foot to work appropriately and not have your shoe overcompensate for certain specifics. Practice these activation sequences before you incorporate your balance exercises.

Place your barefoot on the floor in an inline lunge single leg position. Activate the muscles on the bottom of your foot by slightly gripping the floor and pretending to spread your foot out. Simultaneously squeeze and activate the muscles in your pelvic floor (like you are doing a Kegel exercise) and hold these two squeezes without straining and while maintaining breathing through the diaphragm for about 5 seconds. Release and repeat.

Exercises are listed in order of difficulty. Do not advance

yourself to the next exercise until you have mastered Exercise 1 without any pain.

Exercise 1: Balance Vector Training Single Leg, Vectors 1, 3, and 5

Begin standing single leg with the foot placed firmly on the floor and your core engaged. Vector 1 is when the non-balancing leg is held directly in front of your body, Vector 3 to the side of your body, and Vector 5 behind your body.

The idea is to hold in each balance Vector for 30, 45, or 60 seconds making sure to unload the movement between each balance vector. Do not advance to a form pad or Bosu until all three Vectors become easy.

Exercise 2: Single Leg Balance on Foam Pad, Vectors 1, 3, and 5

Exercise 3: Single Leg Balance on Bosu, Vectors 1, 3, and 5

Exercise 4: Single Leg Balance with Plyo Toss with blue pad and then Bosu

This exercise adds a little bit of reaction time to the balance training. Begin standing single leg with your foot firmly on the ground and your core engaged.

Toss the ball to a trampoline or even your friend and catch it when it comes back to you.

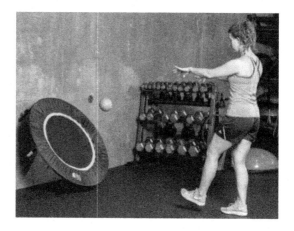

Advance to Single Leg Mini Squat on Bosu, Vectors 1, 3, and 5

Begin single leg on the Bosu and slightly bend your knee and sit into your glutes. Make sure the knee stays behind your toe and that your VMO engages pushing your knee outward a little. Here is an example of a single leg mini squat on the Bosu in Vector 1. Vector 3 will be the same squat with your non-working leg towards your side and Vector 5 would be the same squat with the non-working leg behind you.

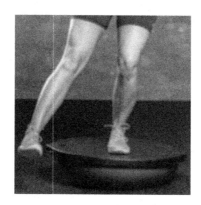

9.2.3 INCREASING CARDIOVASCULAR ENDURANCE

Many of your rehabilitation exercises are focused on strength and balance but gaining back your endurance is going to be a big challenge. The effects of anesthesia can linger in your system for a few days and can affect people very differently. The overall trauma of the surgery alone is enough to shock your system, and with your body focused on healing it isn't going to conserve a lot of energy left for endurance-based activity. With that being said be cautious with building back your endurance. Your progressions are going to be based on pain tolerance so make sure that you only increase your duration a little bit each week in order to avoid pain and swelling. Give your body time to react and get used to moving more.

It would be best to choose low impact movements like a stationary bike or elliptical at first. Start off slow with very little resistance. Work your way up from 2 minutes to 5, 10, and 15 minutes very slowly increasing the resistance only as it starts to feel easy. If you have pain that day, rest. Listen to your body. When you gain more stamina and when your gait patterns have returned to normal it is okay to start walking for longer periods of time. Do not go on long walks until you have gained enough strength and range of motion to walk without a limp. If you do too much walking or activity while your gait patterns are altered it can cause you pain in other places like your feet, back, or hips.

Again, make sure that you start off slowly with your walking. Start with 2 minutes and make your way up to 5, 10, and 15 minutes. Do not walk too fast. It is much better for the biomechanics of your body to walk a little slow using the correct gait patterns than trying to power walk. In terms of biomechanics and avoiding dysfunction, power walking is very bad. Walking is preferred somewhere flat and safe for your knees. Find a spot that has grass or a cushioned track so that you aren't walking on concrete which can be very unforgiving. It is also better to go on a walk somewhere versus walking on a treadmill. Treadmill walking causes people to choose the wrong speed for their gait pattern which will lead to more compensations in posture, form, and ultimately pain. The belt of the treadmill also produces a small force allowing your gait pattern to change. It is almost pointless to practice walking on the treadmill because it will not translate into proper walking form on normal ground.

Athletes like to be challenged. All of this slow walking can start to take a toll on you mentally. It's not a challenge and it's not exciting. Just remember how important it is to properly gain back stamina and do it progressively so that you can avoid setbacks. But in saying all of that it's also imperative to maintain your athletic abilities. In order to truly challenge your cardiovascular system, incorporating interval sprints are a great option. Interval sprints won't be endurance-based but will mostly be a great challenge to help get your heart rate up and help you to stay in great shape and burn fat. Battle ropes are my favorite tool for this. Start off seated on a bench or stability ball so that you avoid trauma and force on the knee. As fast as you can, slam both ropes to the ground as hard as possible. Start off with shorter durations like 15 seconds and do 4 or 5 sets. As this gets easy progress into 30 seconds and increase your sets accordingly. It will be awhile before you can run again, so modified battle rope slams will be a great way to challenge yourself until that day comes.

9.2.4 INCREASING CORE AND GLUTES STRENGTH

During physical therapy you will mostly be working on muscle in the leg that affects the knee. This is good but the entire body is connected and it's vital to be doing everything you safely can to progress yourself. The core and glutes seem to be neglected in many ACL rehabilitation programs. With decreased activity after injury and surgery, you will lose strength in the core and glutes just like you will in your leg.

These muscles affect the performance of an athlete in so many ways. Many studies reveal that weak core musculature and weak glutes contribute to injury risk as well as low back pain. During any sport there are many rapid changes in direction. While the feet and legs are integral to produce these motions so is your core. Every movement uses the core and the dynamic abilities of the core to translate and transmit forces which help athletes to be protected from injury and to be more powerful and explosive.

While it will be difficult to do planks for a while there are still things you can incorporate to strengthen your core in the meantime.

Exercises are listed in order of difficulty. Do not advance yourself to the next exercise until you have mastered Exercise 1 without any pain.

Exercise 1: Stability Ball Crunches and Stability Ball Oblique Crunches

Begin seated on the ball and roll down a little bit allowing your low back to be supported but also where you feel resistance on your core. Engage your core muscles and slowly lift up on the ball. Don't bend your spine too much; make sure the bend comes from your hips. Perform the same motion for the oblique only instead of coming straight up in the center, come up to the right side and to the left side, alternating.

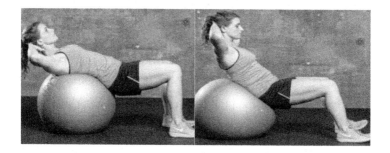

Exercise 2: Modified Cable Woodchoppers on Ball – standing or seated based on recovery/pain

Begin seated on a ball (or standing with your legs slightly wider than hip width apart) and grab the rope with both hands. Pull across and down your body diagonally using your core. Slowly release back to starting position keeping tension.

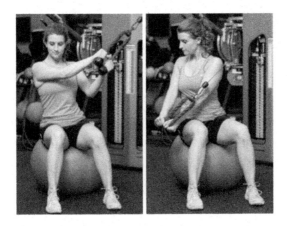

Exercise 3: Modified Plank, and normal Plank

Begin on the floor with your forearms shoulder width apart and your toes on the ground. Lift up into a plank position squeezing your glutes, core, and shoulder blades while breathing. Modify by performing the same move on your knees. Make sure the knees are farther behind your hips versus directly underneath them. Advance up to the normal plank as tolerated by pain and strength.

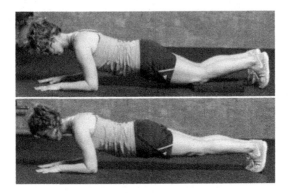

Exercise 4: Stability Ball Bridges

Begin seated on the ball and roll out to a bridge position with your upper back on the ball and your legs and hips out in front of you. Squeeze your glutes and slowly lower your hip down and bring the right back up to the starting point. Make sure that you are only moving your hips up and down. Your body shouldn't move forward or side-to-side, and your feet and upper back shouldn't move at all.

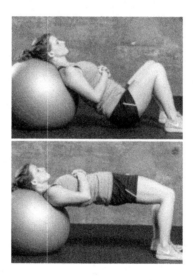

Exercise 5: Modified Side Plank, Side Plank, and Side Plank with Abduction

Start on your side with your elbow directly underneath your shoulder. Your body should be in a straight line with your knees bent and your feet back behind the rest of your body. Hold this positive for 30 seconds on each side and advance your time as you gain strength. After 60 seconds on each side becomes easy you can progress by holding the same position and lifting your top like up and down 15 times like a clam shell. Progress by going from the knees to the feet in the plank and either for a length of time or add in the top leg raise for extra challenge.

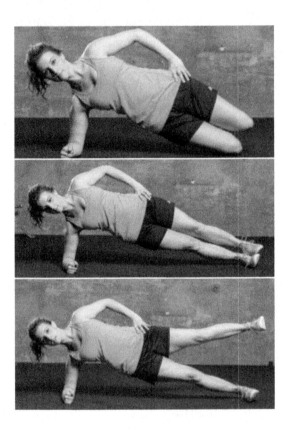

9.2.5 SAMPLE REHAB PROGRAMS

These are suggested strengthening programs to go along with what you are doing in physical therapy. Do not do any exercises if they cause pain and be very slow with the tempo you perform each exercise. Slow and controlled is the goal during this phase of rehab so that you can decrease sheer forces on the knee and increase the stability at your muscles. Do not perform any exercises if they contradict limitations that your doctor prescribed to you. Do not progress to the next phase of exercises until the first phase in pain free and feels easy. If you only have a few physical therapy visits covered by insurance these strength workouts are a great way for you to get more in.

First Phase of Rehab 2 – 6 weeks	2-3 times per week
Exercise	Sets/Reps
Single Leg Hamstring Curl (band)	3/12 or 3/15
Standing Cable Extension	3/12 or 3/15
Standing Cable Flexion	3/12 or 3/15
Standing Cable Abduction	3/12 or 3/15
TKE's	3/12 or 3/15
Single Leg Balance Vectors 1, 3, 5	3/12 or 3/15
Stability Ball Crunches	3/12 or 3/15
Stability Ball Oblique Crunches	3/12 or 3/15
Stationary Bike	5 to 15 minutes

Second Phase of Rehab 6-14 weeks	2-3 times per week
Exercise	Sets/Reps
Single Leg Hamstring Curl (machine)	3/12 or 3/15
Standing Cable Extension	3/12 or 3/15
Standing Cable Flexion	3/12 or 3/15
Standing Cable Abduction	3/12 or 3/15
Eccentric VMO Step Down	3/12 or 3/15
Stability Ball Hamstring Curls	3/12 or 3/15
Lateral Tube Walking	3/12 or 3/15
Cable Woodchoppers on Ball	3/12 or 3/15
Modified Plank on Knees or Normal Plank	3/ 30 sec
Single Leg Balance Vectors 1, 3, 5 on balance pad or bosu	30 seconds, advance up to 45 and 60 seconds
Stability Ball Glute Bridges	3/12 or 3/15
	3/12 or 3/15
Stationary Bike or Elliptical	10 to 30 minutes

Third Phase of Rehab 14-24 weeks	2-3 times per week
Exercise	Sets/Reps
Single Leg Hamstring Curl (machine)	3/12 or 3/15
Step up to Balance	3/12 or 3/15
Single Leg Ball Wall Squat	3/12 or 3/15
Lateral Step up to Balance	3/12 or 3/15
Eccentric VMO Step Down	3/12 or 3/15
Stability Ball Hamstring Curls	3/12 or 3/15
Lateral Tube Walking	3/12 or 3/15
Side Lunge	3/12 or 3/15
Normal Plank on ball or bosu	3/ 30 sec
Single Leg Balance Vectors 1, 3, 5 on blue pad or bosu with plyo toss	30 seconds, advance up to 45 and 60 seconds
Single Leg Bosu Mini Squat Vectors 1, 3, and 5	3/12 or 3/15
Stability Ball Glute Bridges	3/12 or 3/15
Side Plank with Abduction	3/12 or 3/15
Stationary Bike or Elliptical	10 to 30 minutes

The return to function phase of rehabilitation is meant to get you back to your strength levels so that when it's time to integrate total body movements like squats, deadlifts, running, etc. your body will be strong enough to handle the loads and efficient enough not to have compensations on the surgical leg. If the exercise moves begin to feel easy you can increase the number of or repetitions or you can start to add load to the moves by adding 5, 10, and 15 pound dumbbells or kettlebells for extra resistance. Again, we want to get your strength levels as close to normal as possible before beginning any total body movements. The harder you work during this phase of rehab the quicker you will be able to run and jump. It is okay to perform these moves on your uninjured leg because we also want to address strength and compensations in that leg too. But it would be beneficial to focus primarily on the weak surgical leg until strength levels become more even.

9.3 RETURN TO SPORT

After many months of hard work, it's time to advance yourself from gaining strength and function back to your legs and core and into more sport specific training methods in order to prepare your body for your sport or sports of choice. The three most important goals in this last phase of rehabilitation are increasing reaction time, change of direction, landing mechanics, and deceleration training, and sport specific training. This section can also be used for ACL injury prevention methods after advancing through the Return to Function phase in Section 9.2. Make sure to address any weaknesses in the Return to Function phase before pursuing the Return to Sport phase so that all muscle compensation issues have been addressed. This will allow for the body to safely and efficiently prepare for competition by reinforcing proper movement patterns during acceleration, deceleration, jumping, landing, and change of direction movements. After surgery and even after compensating for knee valgus or over-pronation at the foot for a while with no injury, the body can use these mechanics improperly allowing greater injury incidence rates. Going through the Return to Function phase completely first can eliminate these improper muscle firing patterns before taking them into more complex movements.

Many surgeons have different timelines for athletes returning to sport. In some cases athletes are released as soon as six months after their ACL reconstruction. New research on these guidelines comes out every year and we are finding that in most cases a longer recovery makes for a smaller likelihood of re-injury. In fact, "Re-injury risk was reduced by 51% for each month after nine months of post-op recovery for return to sports" *Br. J Sports Med 2016*. It is important to listen to your surgeon's recommendations for recovery timelines because every patient is different, but it is highly recommended to make a timeline appropriate to your skills and abilities, as well as taking your time to ensure that you make a full recovery instead of returning to sport too early. It is not worth the increased risk of injury. Be patient and give your body the time it needs to heal and prepare itself for re-entry to athletics. Despite what many athletes believe, ACL reconstruction recovery is not always a guarantee that you will return to the same level of activity as before surgery. Recent studies show a "55% return to competitive sports following ACL Reconstruction Surgery"

Br. J Sports Med 2014. This is why it is essential to take your time and focus 100% on rehabilitation and recovery.

9.3.1 INCREASING REACTION TIME, CHANGE OF DIRECTION, LANDING MECHANICS, AND DECELERATION TRAINING

With pain, injury, or surgery the body will learn to compensate in order to conserve energy and try to maintain efficiency. Without challenging your reaction time the body will slowly lose its advantages to reacting quickly until you retrain those muscles. It's not only a muscular phenomenon; there are tiny receptors in your ACL and some surrounding ligaments and tissue that communicate with your central nervous system to let your body know feedback about where it is in space and where to move next. Again, pain, injury, and surgery will cause you to be more sedentary decrease use of some of these capabilities. We now have to re-teach the body how to react quickly to different stimuli. In Section 9.2.2. you regained your balance skills which will come into play during this part of your training.

It is best to start off with this slow, controlled, and on two legs until this becomes easy and progressions will help you to get faster and work single leg to challenge yourself even more. The recommended exercises in this section are 4 square jumps, 4-way change of direction sprints, and box jump landings. There are of course many different drills to use for these types of sports training and injury prevention methods and after advancing through these drills feel free to research more that could work for you and your sports team. These are the basic movements that every athlete should be practicing at minimum so it will give you a good idea of if your training programs provided to your team are beneficial. Hiring a qualified speed, agility, and quickness coach is a great tool to prepare yourself and safely learn more drills once you advance from these.

For the 4 square jumps, use rope, tape, or cones to outline a cross like a plus sign. Give yourself enough room to jump and move around so make sure that the cross is about 2 or 3 feet long. Standing over the cross it should look like 4 different squares. Start off with both feet and slowly jump clockwise around the cross, counterclockwise, diagonally, and even have a partner shout out which square to jump to. As this becomes easier increase your speed and when that becomes easy you can progress into the same exercise single leg. Start of slowly and eventually progress into a much quicker pace.

The 4-way change of direction sprints can be easily preformed on a soccer field, volleyball court, or basketball court. Make sure you find somewhere with lines on the field or create your own lines with cones or ropes. You can start off with a shorter distance sprint, maybe 5 to 15 yards, and with increased endurance then increase the distance between to change up the drill. Start out by simply running sprints or suicides between the lines or cones but make sure you run in all four directions; forwards, backwards, and both sides. When you have mastered running sprints in all four directions make it harder by forcing a change of direction when you get to each cone. Sprint to cone 1 and veer to the right. Sprint to cone two and veer to the left. Sprint to cone three and turn a 180-degree turn and sprint to the next cone. To make it even harder, have a partner call out which direction you change to at each cone right as you are approaching on it.

Box jump landings are going to be the most beneficial for athletes who jump a lot like in volleyball and basketball. Take a box either 12", 18", 24", or 36" and begin the movement on top of the box. Jump down off the box and onto the ground making sure that you land efficiently with your feet neutral under the hips, no inward movements at the knees or feet, and without any wobbling around. Try to land softly and use your feet and your core to brace the impact of the landing. Your landing form should look very similar to your squat form. Begin practicing on the ground by just jumping forwards and landing softly and securely. When that becomes easy, begin the box jump landings with a shorter box and increase the number of reps and the height of the box as you progress.

9.3.2 SPORT SPECIFIC

The sport specific training phase will implement everything from the 9.3.1 Section, but now we can customize the training to each individual sport. Different version of sprints in all 4 directions can be done while dribbling a basketball or soccer ball. Basketball players can take rebounds or multiple passes in a row coming from different directions in order to mimic real game time movements. Volleyball players could practice hits coming quickly and coming from all directions. Remember, sport specific training should replicate the real game time experience for the athlete so they are prepared for a real game. Speed ladders are a great way to incorporate speed and quickness training with sport specific training. Run through the speed ladder sideways and be ready to catch a rebound, field a ball, or take off dribbling and shooting. Many combinations can be used so it is best to work with a strength and conditioning coach or speed, agility, and quickness coach. These qualified coaches will help integrate safe and effective programs for athletes at any level to return to sport or prepare for the upcoming season.

Remember that the higher prevalence for ACL tears in men is during the ages of 21-30 where they are more than likely playing pickup sports without warming up or even preparing for the season. Preparing for your sport with sport specific drills can help you to decrease injury during game time when you are going to be more aggressive and not hold anything back. Even after completion of physical therapy and being cleared to return to sport, it is highly advised to hire a skilled speed agility quickness coach or strength and conditioning coach to implement a structured training program to prepare you for sport. If there is any difference in strength or reaction time from one leg to the other you are going to be more prone to re-injury, and remember, because you already tore your ACL you now have a 1 in 50 chance of re-injury. Be safe, be smart, and most importantly be careful and do not advance yourself too quickly, even if you get the clearance.

10

ACL INJURY PREVENTION

Because almost 70% of ACL injuries are non-contact in nature, preventative training programs can have a huge impact on decreasing initial injury and on decreasing rate of re-injury among athletes who have already torn their ACL. Addressing compensations in the individual athlete is key in preventing ACL injury and many athletes have completely different movement patterns and compensations. The female athlete in particular is more prone to ACL injury and an effective neuromuscular training program will dramatically decrease ACL injury risk when applied.

The absolute best way to test for ACL injury risk is to have a trained professional take video of you performing various moves like landing from a jump then immediately jumping forward on one leg. If you are training to return to your sport after an ACL surgery I highly recommend finding a professional in your city who can conduct these screenings and assess your individual injury risk. Try finding a physical therapist, athletic trainer, and strength and conditioning coach specializing in ACL injury prevention and if you are having trouble finding someone in your city please contact me directly off of my website and I will refer you to someone local that you can trust.

Working with a specialist on a custom injury prevention program can dramatically decrease your risk of tearing your ACL but please note that it is not a 100% guarantee. Many factors contribute to ACL injury and unfortunately no matter how much training and injury prevention work is done it still doesn't totally eliminate risk of an ACL tear. Sometimes the body just cannot move in the ways we try to play our sport or a hard hit can force the tear; whatever the case always know that the work you do preventing ACL injury is going to make you a better athlete regardless of your ACL fate. And if you do tear your ACL you are now part of an involuntary family of the most resilient and humble athletes in the world so take your setback and turn it into your most prideful learning and growing experience.

When I first began my ACL journey, my doctor never informed me of the increased risks for ACL tears in 12-17 year-old female athletes or the increased risk of suffering another ACL tear after having your first. This information wouldn't have changed my mind about training for soccer and my goals of making the high school soccer team but it certainly would have changed my approach and made me realize the importance of rehabilitation and injury prevention methods. It most certainly would have motivated me to hire a knowledgeable professional to decrease my injury risk.

That is my goal with this book; to provide others with detailed information that I didn't know when I first when through the surgeries. Everyone who tears their ACL should be aware of their increased risk of re-injury and use the knowledge and guidance from this book to seek out and hire professionals for your youth teams or for your individual skills training. This is the only way we are going to prevent ACL injuries. You do not have to end up like me!

Many of the common compensations for athletes regarding ACL tear are addressed in Chapter 3 and can be corrected with the basic ACL rehabilitation program provided to you in Chapter 9. These compensations occur from anatomical, environmental, hormonal, and structural factors some of which cannot be changed. When there are structural problems effecting muscle patterns, the athlete will learn to be efficient and compensate for these movements using other muscles.

Over time, this leads to increased force at the knee joint, and when corrected, can change the positioning of the knee during athletic movements from creating extra force and improper hazardous mechanics to decreasing tension at the knee and reinforcing or relearning safe mechanics to prevent further stress and injury to the joint. It might seem weird to work on ACL rehabilitation before actually having an ACL tear but by strengthening the same muscles that are weakened after surgery some biomechanical problems causing ACL injury can be fixed. It would be absolutely best to hire a biomechanics expert or highly regarded strength and conditioning coach or athletic trainer to analyze your gait patterns and design a custom program for you, but if budget and resources are a problem, the suggested exercises in Chapter 9 are a great place to start.

Following the protocol for ACL rehab, start with the Return to Function Section in 9.2 and work your way up from there based on your strength levels. This program can be followed in to the Return to Sport section which will better prepare your athlete for reaction time, change of direction, and sport specific movements which when unprepared are major causes of ACL injury.

Because hormonal and structural differences in athletes are somewhat unchangeable like levels of estrogen and the Q angle; the main focus of your prevention training will be around gaining strength and balance to the weaker muscles involved in the Return to Function and Return to Sport sections of ACL rehab and correcting over pronation at the foot, knee valgus, and leg dominance. Strengthening the glutes, hamstrings, quadriceps in particular the VMO, abductors and core; and by increasing balance, proprioception, and reaction time the athlete will have a much stronger foundation for sports and will have a much less likely chance to sustain any type of injury. Female athletes in particular should focus on hamstring, glute, and abductor strength in the lower body.

The best way to test your likelihood of ACL injury is by doing specific movement screenings with a trained professional but for purposes of this book and athletes trying to incorporate an at home program I have simplified this into a basic squat test. This test will not show your risks during landing and decelerating but if you do have knee valgus or over pronation at the foot correcting the issues will help to decrease your likelihood of having poor landing mechanics as usually the way you squat is also the way you land from a jump. By performing a basic squat, we can see if you have over pronation at the foot and knee valgus. Both of which are very common in the female athlete, athletes who sit a lot, and athletes with weak hips and tight calves.

Begin by placing each foot underneath your hips. Perform a full range of motion squat by dropping your hips back and lowering them to the floor. Have a partner watch your feet and your knees separately. Do not try to correct your form. It is important to see what the body naturally does in the squat. Do you see the inside of the feet rolling inward or downward? This view is best seen from behind the athlete. Note the picture on the right, and watch as the foot may or may not change positions throughout the motion of the squat. Make sure the athlete does about 10 squats so you can see multiple repetitions.

Do the knees move inward while squatting? This view is best seen from in front of the athlete. Note the picture on the left, the two-legged squat has good alignment of the knees while squatting and no knee valgus but the photo on the bottom shows where the knees have knee valgus and are caving in. By testing the athlete is a single leg manner you will have the ability to compare each leg and make sure there are no leg dominance issues or deviations from one leg to the other. Remember any compensation from one leg to the other cause an increased risk of injury.

Only perform the single leg testing on an athlete that is capable of doing so. If you would like to take photos or a video it would allow you to step back and watch more slowly in order to recognize the deviations. If you notice the feet rolling inward then there is an over pronation problem and if the knees roll inward there is a knee valgus problem. The good news is that these problems are interrelated and by performing the ACL rehab in Chapter 9.2 and 9.3 it is possible to strength the muscles associated with these compensations and decrease their effects on your body.

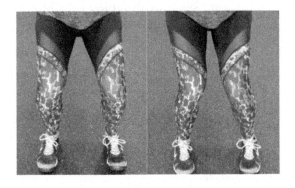

Left: Normal Right: Knee Valgus

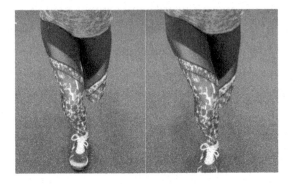

Left: Single Leg Squat Normal Right: Single Leg Squat with Knee Valgus (notice the compensations at the hip, knee, and foot)

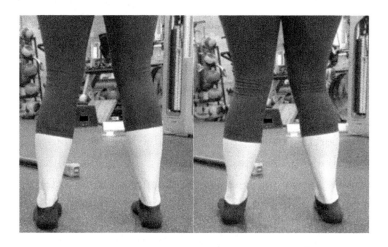

Left: Normal Pronation at Foot Right: Over Pronation at Foot

If you are suffering from leg dominance as a female athlete or leg dominance because of your ACL operation there are many strength training techniques to apply in order to increase strength in the non-dominant leg. In addition to your rehabilitation program make sure that you are doing extra repetitions on your weaker non-dominant leg. You can gain strength in phases by first increasing the repetitions on that leg in order to increase your endurance. I like to perform single leg moves to specifically target the non- dominant leg. Single Leg Step Ups, Lunges, Side Lunges, Single Leg Side Step Ups, Single Leg Hamstring Curls, Single Leg Deadlifts, Bulgarian Spilt Squats, Single Leg TRX Squats. When focusing on leg dominance issues I also perform some workouts only on the weaker less dominant leg so that it can catch up to the stronger dominant side. After increasing your repetitions to 20 reps, it's time to switch your program up and increase your resistance and decrease your reps. Try doing some of the same moves holding a heavy dumbbell or kettlebell and focus on repetitions of 8 to 12. Again, the main focus will still be the non-dominant leg so perform some of your workouts only on that leg until your strength becomes more even.

Through out your training program make sure that you are incorporating balance exercises on the non-dominant leg as well. Balance exercises should always be progressed based on time so start out with a single balance on the floor for 30 seconds and when that is easy move up to 45 seconds and 60 seconds. Then you can progress based on uneven surfaces so select a foam pad or Bosu to stand on following the same time based protocol. When your balance and strength levels are equal on both legs then and only then should you start progressing your rehabilitation into more complex movements like running, landing mechanics, deceleration and change of direction drills, and sport specific training. This protocol might take you longer with the rehabilitation process but it will ensure that you have less compensations resulting from your surgery and a decreased risk of injury regarding issues with leg dominance.

After completing portions of the rehabilitation program, it is great to redo your squat test in order to see if you have made any changes. Look for the same two problems and compare to your old video to see if you have made any improvements. Do not advance into Section 9.3 until you have corrected the over pronation and knee valgus. If you are strong and work hard at these exercises, it shouldn't take you long to move forward. When the compensations regarding your knee valgus, over pronation at the foot, and leg dominance are gone, you can now advance yourself into the Return to Sport phase of training. After going through a strength program to help fix muscle imbalances and compensations, the female athlete will highly benefit from regular ACL injury prevention training. It is best to start training programs focusing on landing mechanics, safe change of direction, and safe deceleration moves at least six weeks before the season starts. Studies have shown that ACL injury prevention programs have helped to decrease ACL injuries in female soccer players but not in female basketball players. This is important for female volleyball and basketball players because their specific warm up before games and practice should involve selected landing mechanics drills and ACL specific prevention moves instead of shooting around on the court. This could make a major change in the statistics for these athletes.

The best way to incorporate sport specific training for ACL injury prevention is to mimic the moves that will be performed in your sport. Practice changing direction moves on the same court, field, turf, or playing surface that you will be playing on. Basketball and volleyball athletes should focus on jumping and landing mechanics. All athletes should focus on decelerating from a sprint safely and making that harder by decelerating from a sprint going directly into a change of direction. Reference the Return to Sport section in 9.3 for specifics on moves to incorporate. Exercises like these should be implemented into all training programs for any youth or teen level sport. If your team doesn't practice changing directions while sprinting or any side-to-side motions involving sprinting or speed ladders, then there is a problem with training methods. The training program should mimic moves involved in the sport and there is no sport where the athletes remain in one direction the entire time. Again, research and hire an appropriate local coach who can customize these moves for you or your entire team. It is worth the investment. By better equipping our athletes with corrective strength training programs to decrease structural and anatomical problems affecting their biomechanics and preparing them with sport specific training, ACL injuries can be decreased dramatically. It's time to make a change and work harder on the prevention side in order to improve the way we approach ACL surgeries and ACL injury prevention methods.

Take home message

- ACL injuries can be reduced by proper strength training programs and addressing movement compensations that occur in individual athletes.
- By preparing athletes for their sport including jumping, landing, deceleration, and change of direction they will have a stronger foundation and muscle memory preparing them for safer movements and decreased risk of injury.
- Basic ACL rehabilitation is a great way to increase strength and balance in muscles that might be atrophied after surgery or just weak, causing more efficient movement patterns at the lower body decreasing risk of injury or re-injury.
- By learning the differences of a female athlete compared to a male we can work together to ensure that female focused strength training and injury prevention programs are available around the country.

11

SURVIVING 7: THE FINAL CUT

The hardest part of this journey hasn't been the surgeries themselves; the pain is temporary but the loss of sport, athletics, and movement short term and long term is much more gut-wrenching. This causes the mental struggle, the debate inside your head trying to find the positives in all of the negativity you are dealing with. The mental struggle can turn temporary physical limitations into long term insecurities and demons. The hardest part of this journey has been not allowing all of these surgeries to define me.

People associate themselves with different identities based on their families, religions, passions, cities, jobs, and sports. As a young girl, I was the soccer chick who quickly became that girl with all the surgeries or that girl in the knee brace. When I went off to college I was able to put those labels behind me and create a new identity for myself. An identity associated with knowledge, exercise science, and the compassion to change people's lives but what's funny is not everyone believed that identity. Even family members thought I was choosing the wrong path or focusing on the wrong things; but, I had to trust myself enough to know that even though there was no such thing as a job title of an ACL Specialist, if I followed my heart I would make it happen. I had to learn that the most important part of my journey is creating my own definition of my own identity for myself because the only person's opinion that matters is my own. Upon graduation from college I wanted to do everything I could to forget about my surgeries and not allow my surgeries and my knees to define me. But through all of this the surgeries have resurfaced again in order to teach me my most important lesson. By learning from my journey, I now know I define myself; not my surgeries. I can create a way to spread my passion and knowledge to help others avoid having a journey like mine. I define myself, not my scars, not my knees. They are pieces of me; struggles that I have endured and because of them I am so strong. I am equipped to have the confidence and the conviction to make an impact in the world of knees. Because of my surgeries, I appreciate having a healthy life and I know with absolute certainty that whatever comes across my path in the future, I will conquer it beyond all odds.

Surviving 7 has taught me that I define myself through my own thoughts and views. I have the power to change my life with any choice I make and I hold the power to change my thoughts so that I can control my outcomes. *Surviving 7* has compelled me to write this book in less than five short months and apply to Physical Therapy school; two things I have always deeply wanted to accomplish but never had the confidence. *Surviving 7* has made me strong. Life is short, and having 7 surgeries before you finish your 27th year is not the best way to spend it. But my mind controls my present happiness, and if these are the only 30 years that I get, I do not regret one moment of them for they have taught me how to be happy, how to create my own success, and how to define my own future for myself not for anyone else. I hope that you approach your ACL surgery with the mindset that you are strong and ready to grow because if you face this head on and allow yourself to be vulnerable and grow and learn through the experience, then you are going to learn some amazing things about yourself. That's what it's all about; growing, learning, and evolving. Without it humans would not exist. Without it, humans would not appreciate existence.

Surviving 7

Jenna M. Minecci

@Jennactive

Jennactive.com

SURVIVOR STORIES

Dialla from Australia - One ACL Surgery
"I had been tackled in my Australian Rules Football match and I heard a popping sound and knew it couldn't be good. A few days later I found out I had ruptured my ACL and considered it one of the worst days of my life. Although hindsight is a wonderful thing, at the time I just burst into tears and cried for a solid two days when anyone tried to talk to me. When people think of me they think of my sporting ability, I've been defined by that most of my life. I was hitting my stride in my football season and had no reason for slowing down and I've never had a major injury. So when this all happened and the reality of how long I would be out for I found it really deflating. I got the ball rolling really quickly and saw my physician, got a rehab program and was referred to a surgeon and had my surgery three and a half weeks later. Although people mean well it really bothered me when they would say 'speedy recovery' when the recovery is 9-12 months. I am three months post-

op at the moment and day 1 seems so far away! I have days when I don't want to leave the house but I still get out of bed and get on with my day. I fear people around my knee, I don't know if it's my trust in people or the trust I have in my knee. I'm very patient and cautious but an extremely motivated person so I have put 'my everything' into this rehab because my biggest fear is that I'll do it again. I still see the beauty in this injury for me personally as I see it as a challenge and a way to become better than I was before the injury, I'm finally hitting my stride with this rehab too and I'm starting to see a light at the end of the tunnel."

Jamil from England – One ACL Surgery

"I tore my ACL in November of 2015 and didn't have my surgery until January 2017. The first few months were extremely difficult! Mainly around feeling sorry for myself! It took me almost two months to get rid of the limp! Eventually I joined a gym and that was a huge turning point! I saw huge progress over the next few months (eight months post-op now). The only frustrating part has been that I've not been able to play the sport (football) that I absolutely love for nearly two years now. Also, within my ACL journey, I've started training to become a qualified geography teacher in London, England. Cut long story short, I've had to basically put my ACL rehab on hold because of the huge work load I have right now! As great as the process has been over the last eight months, right now, juggling my career demands with my ACL rehab has been a big challenge that I have not yet been able to overcome!"

Mimi from New Jersey, United States – Two ACL reconstructions, two meniscus repairs and one meniscectomy -Five surgeries in total and 1 more to go

"In May of 2015, I tore my ACL and meniscus. I had a bucket handle tear so my knee was locked at a 90-degree angle. I went to see a local orthopedic surgeon in my area. He came highly recommended. Because I was in so much pain I just did what he said without doing any research. On June 8th, I went in for an ACL reconstruction and a meniscus repair. When I woke up from surgery he told me everything went great but he wanted to see me in his office in two days. I thought that was normal but later found out it wasn't. Two days later I found myself sitting in his office in terrible pain. He took X-Rays and came back to tell me that the screws holding the graft in place had broken through the bone and I needed another surgery immediately. Two days later I was back at the hospital undergoing a 2nd surgery. After that surgery I was in terrible pain and had a very hard time doing anything let alone rehab. My physical therapist could not get my leg straight no matter how much we worked at it. After eight weeks of rehab without much improvement my surgeon put me on steroids and informed me he was leaving the practice and was handing me over to a different doctor in the practice. Something about the way everything went down made me nervous, so I went for a 2nd opinion. My new doctor was truly a God sent. He immediately saw that something wasn't right and sent for an MRI. The next day I was told that the surgeon had placed my ACL graft too forward and it was impinged on a bone and that was why I wasn't able to straighten my knee. Unfortunately, because of the way my bone reacted the tunnels were so wide and in the wrong place and I needed a bone graft before they could even do reconstructive surgery. So in November I underwent my first bone graft. The doctor used a putty graft because it is less invasive and he thought it would heal well. I spent the next six months trying to gain back strength and stability without an ACL. In May of 2016, I was sent for a CT scan to see how the bone was doing and unfortunately once again I was given bad news, the putty graft did not integrate at all. I then underwent my 2nd bone graft surgery. This one was very invasive and I was in bed rest for ten weeks after. Because of all the complications the doctor was very careful about taking CT scans every six weeks. Throughout this time I was working with a new PT who really pushed me and I was able to gain back a lot of strength but my knee was extremely unstable. It would go out on average three times a day, which made simple activities hard. In March of 2017, my knee went out and usually I could catch it but that night I wasn't able to and I fell. I knew immediately that something was wrong but I was out with friends and didn't want to make a big deal. I sat most of the night in a lot of pain and literally counted the minutes to get home. As soon as I was home I took my leggings off and saw my leg was purple and swollen and I knew I had torn something else. After an MRI was taken I found out I had torn my post lateral corner. My doctor who I really liked and trusted explained that this is not as common as an ACL and that I once again would need to find another doctor because it was out of his capability. He referred me to a doctor who specializes in multi ligament tears. So, in April I found myself sitting in a new doctor's office feeling angry, annoyed and scared! How did a routine ACL reconstruction turn into such a disaster? Well this new doctor explained how the initial mistake spiraled and how at this point he wants multiple scans to make sure everything is aligned properly before we do another surgery. After many scans and tests he felt that before he does the reconstruction I would need an osteotomy (straightening of the bone) I was obviously very nervous to go through another surgery knowing I still wouldn't be done but he explained that without this surgery the grafts would fail and my knee would dislocate. He spoke with several other doctors and was happy to answer all my questions to make sure I was totally comfortable with this surgery. The surgery was done in July 2017 and was harder and more painful than anything I could have imagined. I am still very weak and working so hard to gain back strength. I know that I need to be careful because my knee is so unstable. I have truly learned from this experience not to do anything in a rush. It's ok to ask questions if something doesn't feel right and *don't* ever let any doctor make you feel like you are crazy! If something feels off and a doctor doesn't listen, find one that does!"

Junpei from Japan - One ACL surgery

"I'm a senior playing rugby at a Japanese university. I got hurt in May. I got tackled from both sides and knew straight away something wasn't right. When I found out the news I had torn my ACL, it was very shocking. I am in my last year at university and was pushing for the A-team and now I cannot play this season. I am doing my best to rehabilitate to recover quickly. I want to be able to gain more muscular strength and good performance but it isn't easy. My return is scheduled for March next year. I never realized how hard this would be."

John from Florida, United States – One ACL surgery

"My ACL rupture was a tough and shocking thing to deal with. As an athlete, hearing that you tore your ACL is devastating news. I play Semi-pro football in Florida for the Broward County Barracudas. I had a successful season with just minor injuries. I was selected to play in the All-Star game because of the terrific season that I had. In the 4th quarter of the game, I caught an interception and while returning, I made a hard cut on my right knee and felt a pop with instant pain. After wrapping my knee with an ACE wrap, I was able to drive to the emergency room where an X-Ray was performed. I was told that there were no broken bones or dislocation and I should get an MRI done. I visited my doctor and he tested my knee and said that my ACL was in good shape. I didn't want to take that as an answer. I had an MRI scheduled and the news came back, ruptured ACL. I shed a few tears initially because my success in semi-pro opened more doors for me. Once I had surgery, I started my physical therapy the next day. I've been motivated by focusing on all of the positives that I achieve through my therapy. The only time where I'm not doing some kind of physical therapy is while I'm sleeping. I had a minor setback when I strained my calf muscle but I focus on the outcome, so the calf strained didn't affect me mentally. A major injury like an ACL rupture can be a mental and physical struggle, but if you focus on the small victories then that would help you in your recovery process."

Jennifer from Germany – Three ACL surgeries

"The story behind the scars is so tough, painful, frustrating and beautiful. Taking rest days... sometimes this is the hardest part for us athletes but rest allows our body to heal, to reduce the swelling and for our muscles to recover.

This injury is a true test to see just how strong you are both mentally and physically.

My history:

1st surgery: ACL reconstruction with semitendinosus tendon right knee

2nd surgery: ACL reconstruction with semitendinosus tendon left knee

3rd surgery: Bone grafting right knee

4th surgery: Revision ACL reconstruction with quadriceps

tendon & anterolateral stabilization (modified Lemaire procedure) right knee

I spent one and a half years with my 3rd torn ACL. I was able to stay fit & enjoy exercise w/out it, but I personally felt like it disrupted my active lifestyle somewhat, as far as handball, cycling, & skiing. I re-injured my right knee during a running workout. There was a sudden sharp pain - worse than the initial injury. Bad bone bruising & swelling. After that I was glad to get the surgery, so I wouldn't have to worry about that again. I went to a very skilled surgeon to Berlin & worked hard to rehab. Now my knee feels stronger than it did pre-injury. I do hip/knee exercises to stay strong. Getting back to normal training is the most amazing feeling ever! Sometimes it takes the worst pain to bring out the best. I think it all just depends on personal expectations & finding a top-notch surgeon if surgery is desired. I've seen a lot of friends need 2nd or 3rd ACL surgeries after going to a bad surgeon to start. I would rather wait a few months to get into see the best.

I recommend to everyone with an active lifestyle to get the surgery. The rehab is hard work and painful but in the end worth it!

Many ups and downs but finally it's all over and I am getting back stronger than before. It was really the best thing I ever did. Rehab was a pain but pushed through it. Bottom line surgery isn't always needed, but if it helps a lot!

The rehab is long and needs a lot of commitment and you have to be prepared to do it.

Reading about other people going through the same thing has helped me a lot so I hope this helps someone out there to stay positive and strong!"

***

Sarfina from Malaysia, Golfer – 1 ACL surgery, 1 meniscectomy, possibly 1 more ACL surgery to go

"Monday, Feb 2nd 2015 – Finally feels like I've settled in to this new routine and schedule. A new country, new school, new teammates, new culture. I was scared of the adjustment; it was overwhelming and confusing yet the thought of having the opportunity to be amongst the small percentage of people that get to live out their dream of getting a degree while playing the sport they love so very much was worth it. This is what I dreamed of as a little girl, holding that golf club for the very first time I knew this was what I wanted to do for the rest of my life.

February 3rd 2015 - The day that would change my life forever. The women's golf team consisted of seven talented girls. We had just started with team workouts in preparation for the upcoming spring season. Tuesday the 3rd, was our 2nd training session. As I completed one circuit and moved on to the next all that stood between me and the pull up bar was a wooden box. A harmless light brown box that was situated right under the bar to help us reach a little better. Next thing I know, a very distinct sound and sensation–a pop. Seconds later, came the excruciating pain. The pain is something I cannot put into words even to this day. I was seen by a few Athletic Trainers and a doctor later on that same day and nothing seemed to be amiss. Possible knee sprain someone said. I started rehabilitation a couple days later to strengthen my knee and the muscles surrounding it to make sure I was back to normal by the end of February for our first tournament. About a week later, my coach and I sat down for a chat. This isn't unusual seeing she likes to be involved with what is going on in her player's lives and wants to help make our college experience as smooth as possible. She brings up an MRI. I ask her why and she said just to make sure you're good to go. "We want to be sure," she said.

"You have to be very still; the machine is very sensitive to movement." The radiologist said. 45 minutes later and I had my first MRI of my right knee. Unfortunately, it would not be my last. We waited anxiously for the results, my place on the travel team up in the air because of my unknown condition. Friday evening came around; a few days had passed since the MRI and I get a phone call from my athletic trainer asking me to come in for a chat. This was odd I thought seeing it was almost 5pm. The walk to the training room was surprisingly calming, I took the view in and listened to all the different sounds around me. I wanted to save that image in my mind in preparation for what was to come next. My trainer guided me into one of the offices in the back and had me sit down. He then proceeded to break the news, "I'm afraid you have completely torn your ACL, you are going to need surgery." Those words didn't sink in until later that night. I got to see the MRI report a few days later and it said I had a complete tear of the ACL and an MCL sprain. Here I was all alone with no family in the country, facing the biggest surgery of my life. I did not know what to expect or how I was going to go forward from here. My dreams of a collegiate golf career quickly disappearing right in front of my eyes.

March 5th & 6th – A cloud of white right outside my window. It had not stopped snowing for hours and there was no way I was going to be able to make it to the hospital or get home. I knew it was an outpatient procedure and I would be a fall risk after surgery so it was best to have the surgery pushed. As if he had heard my thoughts from the day before, I get a call from my surgeon at 6:30am on March 5th to tell me that my surgery was going to be postponed to the 6th seeing the storm was finally passing and I would be able to come in. March 6th came around quickly. I had my bags packed and made a final call back home to let my parents know that I was going on. My coach drove me to the hospital bright and early in the morning. We were taken back and I was told to change so they could get my vitals and start an IV. They struggled a little with the IV but 2 pokes later we had one going and I was given some medicine to calm my anxious mind and body. I was then taken back to get my femoral nerve block; I did not feel much at this point because I was very calm and a little out of it from the medicine. They then took me back to the holding area and had me sign a few more forms and confirm the limb that I was having surgery on. My surgeon came in and signed my leg and soon I was off to the operating room.

The pain was so intense it felt like whatever pain medication they gave me wasn't working. I remember

seeing my athletic trainer sitting by my bed and asking me
how I felt. They struggled keeping my pain under control
so I was taken to a recovery room so they could continue IV
pain medication. 2 days later I was discharged and on my
way home. I quickly realized how little I could do
independently and that made me angry because I was so
used to doing things on my own. I didn't want help but I
needed it. I struggled with this a lot throughout the
recovery process. The biggest thing I learned during the
recovery period is you learn who your true friends are. You
truly see who will have your back no matter what happens.
I lost a lot of friends and family during this time and I
grieved hard because I would do anything for these people
yet they didn't feel the same way about me. I rehabbed hard
to try and get back in time for the Fall season. My surgeon
and athletic trainers came up with a plan and we stuck to it.

August 2015 – 5 months post-surgery I played in my first
tournament. I felt great and my knee was doing well, I was
in very little pain and had no swelling. I played great at the
first tournament and my coach and I thought I was ready to
be back. At the very next tournament a couple weeks later,
I could hardly walk, let alone swing a club. The pain was
intense and I was scared. I went in for another MRI as soon
as we got back and to my surprise it came back clear. Many
individuals that I trusted went against me and said I was
making things up or that it was all in my head. My coach
and I decided to take a step back and head back to the
drawing board. I sat out the rest of the season and went
back to the training room to do rehabilitation daily to get
back some of the strength and range of motion that I
had lost.

The pain never stopped but that didn't stop me from working on my game doing my exercises in the training room. I played both Spring and Fall seasons of 2016 in pain but it wasn't until the Fall season where I was so tired of being in constant pain I stood up and asked to see my surgeon. He suspected a meniscus tear and low and behold it was confirmed on an MRI. Knee surgery number 2 was planned for November 2016. I went in not knowing if he would do a meniscectomy or a repair but either way I was ready for the pain to stop. He ended up doing a partial lateral meniscectomy and removed a cyclops lesion. Pain was in my past at this point, I felt like a whole new person. I had to start all over again from square one with range of motion and strength but it was easier to overcome because I knew I had done it before. Then it hit me like a ton of bricks, about 6 months out from surgery I was in more pain than ever before. It started slowly and was not very frequent, I would hurt when my activity level went up but as time went on it progressively became constant and increased in intensity.

Today- I have seen my surgeon twice since September and he believes my graft may have stretched which could be causing my symptoms. I had MRI number 4 done a few days ago and once again was diagnosed with a tear in the lateral meniscus. As I wait for my follow up in less than two weeks I cannot help but think my future remains unclear and I am being forced to change my goals once again. My collegiate carrier is once again up in the air. I am at a fork in the road and there are no signs to help me pick the correct path to go down. I never thought 2 years and 6 months out from my initial surgery I would still be dealing with this problem. However, that is okay, I believe everything happens for a reason and through this injury I have learned who my real friends are, I have learned patience, resilience and grit. It is okay to be scared and confused. It is okay to have good and bad days. My journey may be very different from yours but we all walk down our own paths and there are no guides to show us how to deal with the forks in the road or the barriers along the way. The most important thing that I have learned through all of this is to trust my instinct and trust my body. You know which way to go, you just need to allow yourself to feel and see it. This entire process has been a learning curve for me and I see that now more than ever. My journey may be far from over and it may never be over but the sun continues to rise and as this happens I will put one foot in front of the other and keep walking down my path."

REFERENCES

1) Voskanian, Natalie. "ACL Injury prevention in female athletes: review of the literature and practical considerations in implementing an ACL prevention program." Curr Rev Muskulatoskelet Med. Feb 15, 2013. https://www.ncbi.nlm.nih.gov/pmc/articles/PMC370278 1/

2) Friedberg M.D., Ryan. "Anterior Cruciate Ligament Injury." http://www.uptodate.com/contents/anterior-cruciate-ligament-injury

3) Boden, Sheehan, Torg, Hewett. "Noncontact anterior cruciate ligament mechanisms and risk factors." Sep, 2010. https://insights.ovid.com/pubmed?pmid=20810933

4) Imwalle. Myer. Ford. Hewett. " Relationship between hip and knee kinematics in female athletes during cutting maneuvers: a possible link to noncontact anterior cruciate ligament injury and prevention" Nov. 2009.

https://www.ncbi.nlm.nih.gov/pmc/articles/PMC356524
1/

5) Brophy. Silvers. Gonzalez. Mandelbaum. "Gender Influences: the role of leg dominance in ACL injury among soccer players" June 11, 2010. http://bjsm.bmj.com/content/early/2010/06/01/bjsm.200 8.051243

6) Lenehan EA, Payne WB, Askam BM, Grana WA, Farrow LD. "Long-Term Outcomes of Allograft Reconstruction of the Anterior Cruciate Ligament" Am J Ortho. 2015 May, 4. http://www.mdedge.com/amjorthopedics/article/98945/a rthroplasty/joint-replacement/long-term-outcomes-allograft

7) Wiggins, Grandhi, Schneider, Stan eld, Webster, Myer. "Risk of Secondary Injury in younger athletes after anterior cruciate reconstruction" Am J Sports Med. 2016; Ju; 44(7) https://www.ncbi.nlm.nih.gov/pmc/articles/PMC/55012 45/

ABOUT THE AUTHOR

Jenna obtained her Bachelors of Science in Kinesiology from the University of Tennessee. Additionally, she is an Orthopedic Rehabilitation of the Knee Specialist. She is a certified Strength and Conditioning Specialist through the National Strength and Conditioning Association and a Certified Personal Trainer, Corrective Exercise Specialist, and Performance Enhancement Specialist through the National Academy of Sports Medicine. She holds additional certifications as a Movement and Mobility Specialist through Mobility Wod and a Functional Movement Screen Specialist. Jenna plans to obtain her Doctorate in Physical Therapy. She is very passionate about helping others facing ACL surgery.

For More Information:
www.Jennactive.com
On Social Media
@Jennactive
Email: JMinecci@gmail.com

Lightning Source UK Ltd.
Milton Keynes UK
UKOW01f0639090218
317600UK00014B/353/P